What People Are Sayin

Energetic Anatomy Made Easy

Energetic Anatomy Made Easy is a unique and innovative analysis of the chakras and Traditional Chinese Medicine (TCM). I have mentored Dr. Stuart in her TCM studies for many years. She is one of my best students and I am confident in her work as a TCM practitioner. *Energetic Anatomy Made Easy* is a welcomed insight into both Western yoga and Traditional Chinese Medicine.
Dr. Shiwu Xiao, MD (China), L.Ac., M.S.O.M.

Dr. Laurel Stuart is a graduate of the Canadian Institute of Traditional Chinese Medicine (CITCM). While she was at school she had already shown her talent and interest in combining her longstanding practice of yoga with the ideology of Qi (energy) and the meridians in Chinese Medicine. It is my honor to write this endorsement for her book *Energetic Anatomy Made Easy: Create Better Health Through An Understanding Of Your Chakras and Meridians*.

With years of experience as a yoga instructor and a Traditional Chinese Medicine practitioner, Dr. Stuart has in *Energetic Anatomy Made Easy* perfectly blended her knowledge of the chakras, acupoints, meridians, and internal organs from a physical and energetic point of view. This book is an exceptional practice manual to enrich body, mind, spirit, and soul.
Dr. Xia Cheng, MD (China), R.Ac., Ph.D., Executive Director of CITCM (Canadian Institute of Traditional Chinese Medicine)

I recommend *Energetic Anatomy Made Easy* to help you, the reader, unravel the mysteries of your internal wilderness. Laurel has crafted for you a road map for self-knowledge. Invaluable!

We need all the help we can get on our heroine/hero's quest for wisdom. Good journey to you!

Ana T. Forrest, Co-creatrix of Forrest Yoga

An enlightening, easy read. The introduction really tied things together for me and I returned to it after reading all the chapters. I also really appreciated the appendices with definitions of the jargon unfamiliar to me. As a novice in regard to the concepts the book has provided, I found that the introduction enabled me to best determine my 'take home' — what resonated with me, what could I take into my life's journey even if I never practice yoga, meditate, or ponder on the energy systems that travel through my body. The key aspects from my reading were the beginning pages of each chapter: the three words of each chakra/meridian that provided the foundation (easy to remember); life themes (significance and focus), and most of all the affirmations (my action items). I loved the idea of personalizing each affirmation to make it meaningful and purposeful.

Diane Grant, Clinical Genetics Manager, Anatomical Pathology & Cytopathology

I have known Laurel for many years and she has always been a confident, level-headed individual that is deeply passionate about yoga. She has invested many years in developing her skill, practice, and knowledge of yoga and alternative medicine and is able to explain much of what she does and why in layman's terms to novices and advanced practitioners alike.

I am proud to see that she has taken the initiative to author a book focused on a subject matter that she intimately lives and breathes, in her quest to share the spirit of yoga with the world as a means of grounding oneself, improving self-awareness and healthy living.

Laurel has several years of experience teaching yoga as well, and this has no doubt been a source of strength when she decided to write her yoga book. Her consistent practice of yoga has allowed her the strength and confidence to pursue her dream of alternative medicine, which she is now able to offer as a holistic approach to living a healthy life.

Laurel is good—very good—and I encourage anyone who has but even a passing interest in yoga or alternative medicine to read her book and reach out to her.

Nad Cyrus, Vice President of Information Technology, Cidel Bank & Trust Inc.

Energetic Anatomy Made Easy

Create Better Health through an Understanding of Your Chakras and Meridians

Energetic Anatomy Made Easy

Create Better Health through an Understanding of Your Chakras and Meridians

Laurel Stuart

AYNI
BOOKS

Winchester, UK
Washington, USA

JOHN HUNT PUBLISHING

First published by Ayni Books, 2023
Ayni Books is an imprint of John Hunt Publishing Ltd., No. 3 East Street, Alresford
Hampshire SO24 9EE, UK
office@jhpbooks.com
www.johnhuntpublishing.com
www.ayni-books.com

For distributor details and how to order please visit the 'Ordering' section on our website.

ISBN: 978 1 80341 291 7
978 1 80341 292 4 (ebook)
Library of Congress Control Number: 2022944884

A CIP catalogue record for this book is available from the British Library.

Design: Lapiz Digital Services

UK: Printed and bound by CPI Group (UK) Ltd, Croydon, CR0 4YY
Printed in North America by CPI GPS partners

We operate a distinctive and ethical publishing philosophy in
all areas of our business, from our global network of authors to
production and worldwide distribution.

Contents

We are actually educated into believing that nothing is real beyond what we can perceive with our ordinary senses.
Sogyal Rinpoche

Health Disclaimer

The information presented in this book is for educational purposes only and is solely the opinion of the author. The information in this book is not intended to diagnose, treat, cure, or prevent any condition or disease.

Please seek advice from your healthcare provider for your personal health concerns prior to taking advice from this book.

Preface

This book was created for yoga students. Yoga students who have an interest in learning about energy healing. Yoga students in search of straightforward practices that will deepen their understanding of Western chakra psychology and Traditional Chinese Medicine. This book is a discourse on Western yogic traditions and Taoist wisdoms and a manual on how these wisdoms can be applied to our daily lives in ways that promote well-being.

Each chapter examines a specific chakra and its associated Chinese Medicine organ or organs and meridians. Different chakras and meridian energies overlap in their physiology and anatomy. The energy bodies, unlike our physical body, are subtle and highly fluid. Every chapter in the manual contains comparisons between the chakras and meridians, and activities that nourish the specific energy center and its associated anatomy. Affirmations given throughout the book can be used as written or tailored to address the reader's unique life experiences. The recipes given are meant to stimulate the reader's imagination on how to physically feed both the energetic and physical bodies. The reader may choose to practice the hand mudras while meditating. The yoga sequences can be lengthened or shortened depending on the student's time constraints. Mindful breathing is all that is truly required when practicing the yoga asanas. It is hoped that readers find time at the end of each yoga sequence for savasana.

We are each filled with a rainbow of energies that give depth and meaning to our lives. I am grateful for the wisdom teachers that have passed before me. The teachers that keep the knowledge of the esoteric wisdoms alive. The teachers that pass on the teachings. May this manual be useful to you as you learn to embrace and resonate with all the colors of your internal rainbow.

Aho.

Acknowledgments

There is an African proverb—it takes a village to raise a child.

Without community, family, and friends, *Energetic Anatomy Made Easy* would not be as it exists today.

To Adara Yoga Studio (Barbados) and Passage Studios (Calgary, Alberta), thank you for your assistance in making this book a reality. Most of the photos in this book would not have been possible without the kindness of these two communities.

To my yangster models—Indi McClean, Cyd Cyrus, Carla Boyce, Barry Stuart, Diane Best, and Juliet Stuart, and to my yinster models—Assane Ka, Cindy Sobo, Gord Desautels, Kristin Jostad, Erica Leong, and Lyse Riza, I am eternally grateful for your beauty in these pages. With your help I am able to show the world just a fraction of the beauty and diversity that is found in yoga.

To Ana Forrest, my principal yoga mentor—thank you for enriching my spirit with your teachings and passion. Your work has profoundly influenced my life path and the woman that I am today. I am blessed to have you as a guide.

To my teachers of Traditional Chinese Medicine and yin yoga, I am deeply grateful for the wisdoms you share with me.

To my illustrator Dionne Graham. You did a fantastic job. I am so happy I was able to work with you on this project.

To my friends Cyd Cyrus, Harriette Neblett and Nelson Arsenault. Your support was invaluable to me as I wrote this book. I dearly appreciate you.

To my family, in particular my mum and dad, my uncle Dale, and my brothers—you are my roots. I know I am very fortunate to walk on this planet with you by my side.

And finally to Nellie, my essence—the nurturing vivacious warmth you gave to me, and everyone else around you, will never be forgotten.

Thank you.

Introduction

A WORD ON THE YOGA, THE MERIDIANS, THE ACUPOINTS, AND THE CHAKRAS

Yin and yang are as intertwined in yoga as they are in every aspect of life. In Chinese characters yin is depicted as a hill covered by clouds while yang is depicted as a hill under the rays of the sun. Yin and yang are ways of describing all matter and energy. The qualities associated with yin are more meditative, unhurried, feminine, heavy, and restful. The qualities associated with yang are more active, brisk, masculine, warming, and light.

In Traditional Chinese Medicine the vital substances that make up our body can be classified using yang or yin. Qi (our life force energy) and shen (our spirit) are considered more yang; while blood, body fluids, and our life essence are considered more yin. In Traditional Chinese Medicine the meridians are the pathways or channels that transport the vital substances throughout the body. The entire body is connected by the meridians. The meridians nourish and protect our mental, emotional, and physical health. Acupuncturists use knowledge of the meridians to promote good health and to treat ill health.

In Traditional Chinese Medicine there are several types of meridians. Some meridians run closer to the surface of the body while others are located deeper within. *Energetic Anatomy Made Easy* focuses on the primary meridians and how some of them compare to the chakras of twentieth-century yoga. The chakras in Western yoga are vortices of energy in the body. Each chakra is associated with specific vibrations or frequencies. The health of a chakra affects the physical, mental, and emotional bodies. The health of the physical, mental, and emotional bodies affects the health of the chakras. The primary meridians all have acupoints on the surface of the body. They also travel deeper in the body to connect to specific organs. All but two of the primary channels are bilateral. Acupoints are gateways along the meridians that can improve the health of the meridian and its associated organs.

Acupoints, like the chakras, can be used as focal points during meditation and yoga practice. Stimulating acupoints while practicing yoga allows for an expanded form of energy healing, as compared to practicing yoga alone.

There are two yoga sequences in each chapter of this book—a yang or Forrest-style yoga practice and a yin yoga practice. Both practices are designed to encourage wellness and a stronger understanding of our energetic anatomy. Work with one theme per yoga session. Use the themes to develop a deeper awareness of your energetic body. Fascinate on exploring your inner world using focus and breath.

In our stressful high-paced world, yoga practices comprised of mostly yin qualities have become increasingly popular. In yin yoga, postures are held for anywhere between 1 and 20 minutes. In Forrest yoga, postures can be held for up to a few minutes but are normally held for anywhere between 3 and 10 breaths, depending on the level of the practitioner.

Forrest yoga sessions normally begin with a focus on class intent. Forrest yoga sessions also include abdominal exercises in the warmup section of the class. Forrest yoga asks its practitioners to breathe deeply. It also asks its practitioners that they be willing to *feel* with great honesty for what they are doing in each moment and the energy they are embodying in each posture.

Yin yoga has three basic principles for practice. These are 1) coming into the pose at an appropriate intensity, 2) staying still in the pose—unless there is a need to either reduce or deepen the intensity of the pose, and 3) remaining in the pose for an appropriate length of time, to target specific joints and connective tissues. Yin postures should never feel extremely intense, as these sensations can lead to injury. Yin yoga is a deeply meditative style of practice that allows for a profound release on all levels and physical relaxation.

Stimulating the acupoints given in each chapter can be done prior to, during, or after the yoga sequences. The scope of this book allows for stimulation of acupoints via massage or sound. To stimulate the acupoints using sound, readers will need to invest in sound healing tools such as body tuning forks. These forks look like regular tuning forks, but they are specifically engineered for body tuning. Stimulating an acupoint three times with a tuning fork (letting the vibration of the fork drain into the acupoint) is normally considered sufficient. Do not use a body tuning fork if the sensations it creates feel uncomfortable or do not resonate with you. If using massage, press on each point for approximately 1 minute to start stimulating the acupoints healing energies. Acupoints can often feel sore when massaging. Some acupuncturists use soreness and tenderness to find out which points need extra stimulation. Acupoints that are not sensitive to the touch can still be very useful in treatments.

Chapter 1

The Root Chakra (Muladhara) &
The Kidney Meridian

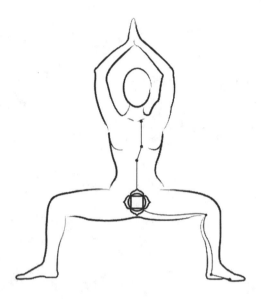

GROUND
ROOT
SUPPORT

I embrace the beauty of my beginnings.

Our root chakra, muladhara, is the energetic base of our existence. Muladhara is located between the anus and the genitals. Its energy connects us to the earth. In Western yoga, muladhara governs our legs, bones, spinal column, perineum, and immune system. It is associated with the building of our cells, and our thoughts and ideas regarding family, community, survival, and support.

Muladhara is most analogous to the kidney organ and meridian in Traditional Chinese Medicine (TCM). The first acupoint on the kidney meridian is located on the bottom of our feet. It is the only acupoint in the 14 major meridians that is located on the sole of our feet. The kidney meridian then rises along the posterior aspect of our inner legs to our coccyx, where it then travels through our lower spine, to connect to our kidneys and urinary bladder. It then ascends through our liver, diaphragm, and lungs, where one branch terminates at the root of the tongue and another branch terminates in our chest, after connecting to the heart. The last acupoint on the kidney meridian is located just beneath our collarbones.

In TCM the kidneys govern our congenital energy; our innate intelligence to live, survive, and prosper. The strength of our memory, our willpower, our bones, and our lower back is strongly associated with the kidneys in Traditional Chinese Medicine.

Healthy root chakra energy allows us to feel comforted, rested, grounded, and secure. With a healthy root chakra our life force is strong. With healthy kidney energy our constitutional energy is strong. Healthy kidney energy supports the other organs of our body and allows for the development and maintenance of a strong body and mind.

Attend to your most basic needs. Honor what is good from your roots.

Home is an inner space; a safe nurturing retreat that allows us the possibility to explore the outer world.

LIFE THEMES

- Feeling nurtured, grounded, and safe
- Fostering healthy solid friendships and tribes
- Overcoming chronic fear as a way of life; learning through fear without being weakened or restricted by it

BALANCED MULADHARA CENTER / HEALTHY KIDNEY ENERGY	IMBALANCED MULADHARA CENTER / DEFICIENT KIDNEY ENERGY
Healthy legs and feet Healthy adrenals and bones Healthy vitality A mindset of abundance and security *NB: The last point is found only within Western yoga.*	Weak legs or bones, adrenal fatigue Lower backache, arthritis, water weight Weak vitality A mindset of fear; an inability to focus due to feeling 'disconnected' Feeling victimized or vulnerable Obsession with material things; hoarders *NB: The last two points are traditionally only found in Western yoga. They are not found in Traditional Chinese Medicine.*

AFFIRMATIONS

1. I am firmly rooted in all my endeavors.
2. I have a community that cares for me.
3. I am worthy of all things beautiful.
4. The earth fully supports me, nourishes me, and nurtures me.
5. My bones are strong and healthy.

Making Affirmations Personal

Affirmations are more powerful when they are believable to you. Tailoring affirmations specifically to your unique life situations makes them more believable.

Here is one way to personalize affirmation 2 from the list above—*My friends Cindy and Arturo care about my well-being.*

Here is a personalization of affirmation 5—*My legs are strong enough for me to take a short walk today.*

YOGA SEQUENCES

GENERAL THEMES

- Practice the yoga sequences in this section with the intention of embracing the energies a healthy home provides. What are some of the energies a healthy home should provide? How do you embody those energies as you practice?
- Are you frequently plagued with feelings of fear? Fear is the emotion most associated with the kidneys. Fear can deeply weaken our kidneys, particularly during infancy and early childhood. Where do you feel fear in your body? Can you breathe into those areas in a way that starts to release or ease that emotion?
- Affirmations such as those mentioned above can be repeated internally during the practice.
- Breathe into your lower dantian (the area below your navel). Place one hand on your lower abdomen and one hand on your lower back. As you inhale, feel the space between your hands expanding. Focus on breathing into your lower dantian throughout your practice.

Beginners: Fascinate on feeling your feet and legs while you practice.

POSES

Tree Pose

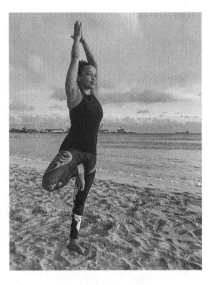

Warrior 1

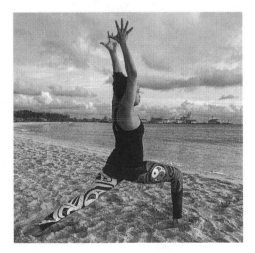

FORREST YOGA SEQUENCE

IDEAS FOR INTENTION

- How do I practice each of these poses in a way that allows me to feel content/grounded/balanced/safe? (Any of these themes can be worked with.) Be open to the question. As you open to the question, your brain starts to work on helping you to find an answer.
- Do I feel grounded in this pose? Am I connected to my feet and my toes?
- Can I feel or acknowledge the strength and solidity of the earth beneath me?

Horse Stance

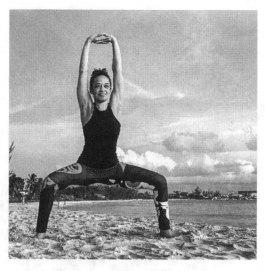

For a longer class, start with: Frog Lifting through Abdominals, Sun Salutations

Pregnant individuals: No abdominal work is permitted during pregnancy. It is also important that your body is well supported in your practice. Use chairs and wall props if you prefer a less strenuous practice. For example, Horse Stance can be practiced while sitting on a chair or Tree Pose can be practiced using a wall for support.

YIN YOGA SEQUENCE AND THE ACUPOINTS

ACUPOINTS

- K3 (Kidney 3) *Supreme Stream*

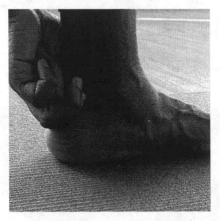

A primary point along the kidney meridian that nourishes all aspects of kidney function in Traditional Chinese Medicine. It can be used with B60 to ground the spirit and create feelings of safety.

Location: In the depression directly behind the highest point of the inner ankle bone.

- B60 (Urinary Bladder 60) *Kunlun Mountains*

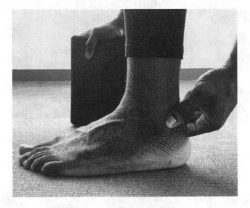

POSES

Dangling

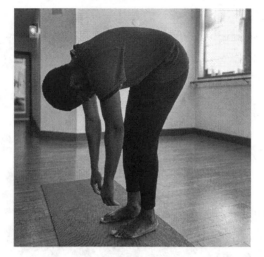

Baby Dragon

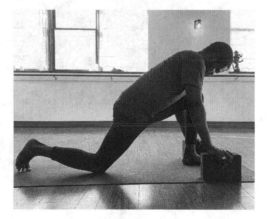

B60 is an important point for clearing pain along the path of the urinary bladder meridian. The urinary bladder meridian starts at the inner eye, runs over the top of the head, then runs along the back of the body on either side of the spine and down the back of the legs to terminate at the little toe. Bladder points are frequently used in TCM to improve spinal and back health. The urinary bladder meridian is intricately connected to the kidney meridian. Coupled with K3 it is commonly used to ground energy. It is contraindicated in pregnancy.

Location: In the depression directly behind the highest point of the outer ankle bone.

- K7 (Kidney 7) *Returning Current*

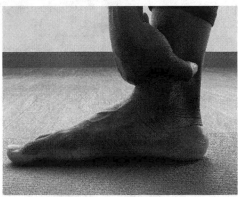

Kidney 7 is the mother point of the kidney meridian. Like a mother to her child, K7 can be used to nurture all aspects of kidney function. K7 helps regulate water metabolism in the body. It is sometimes used in combination with other points to treat edema and sweating disorders.

Location: Measure the length from the knuckle of the index finger to the tip of the index finger (this measurement equals two cun). K7 is located 2 cun above K3, directly in front of the Achilles tendon.

Wall Caterpillar

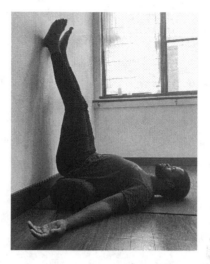

For a longer class, end with: Toe Squat, Reclining Twist

Pregnant individuals: Replace Baby Dragon with Dragon Flying High. Ensure there is no pressure on the abdomen while performing Dangling. Dangling can be practiced with the hands resting on the wall for support as you bend forward. Elevate your back and head in Wall Caterpillar as necessary with pillows and/or bolsters. If it is uncomfortable, omit Wall Caterpillar altogether.

RECIPES

BEET BOOST
Serves 2

The earthy red color of this smoothie is characteristic of root chakra energy. Red is the color most associated with the root chakra. Black is also associated with the root chakra. Black is the color associated with the kidneys in Chinese Medicine. Studies have found beets are a good source of manganese, a mineral that may be useful in keeping bones healthy. In Chinese Medicine beets are helpful for nourishing the blood. Blood is partially governed by the muladhara chakra. Mint is used in TCM to help fight off colds, so this smoothie is good for the throat chakra and lungs as well as the first chakra.

- Medium-size red beet, peeled and sliced
- 3 cups freshly squeezed orange juice
- 1 small handful of mint

Blend the beet, orange juice, and mint until smooth. Serve immediately.

MOLASSES ROOIBOS TEA
Serves 2

Molasses is flooded with B vitamins. It is a highly nourishing food that may help reduce the effects of stress on the body. Cinnamon coupled with the creaminess of coconut milk makes for a comforting texture and aroma.

- 1 teabag rooibos tea
- 1½ cups hot water
- 2 cups warm coconut milk
- Pinch of salt

- 1 teaspoon (tsp) molasses
- 2 dashes of allspice, 2 dashes of cinnamon
- 1 tablespoon (tbsp) brown sugar

Boil the hot water. Let the water cool for 1 minute, then steep the tea for 5 minutes. Pour the tea into a high-speed blender with warmed coconut milk, sugar, salt, molasses, and spices. Blend well. Sprinkle with cinnamon. Serve hot.

BAKED COU COU AND SALT FISH
Serves 3

Foods for the root chakra are normally heavy, comforting, and grounding. Be mindful that what is most comforting to another may not be what is most comforting for you. Cou cou and flying fish is the national dish of Barbados. Barbados is my birth tribe. Nothing spells comfort for me like a bowl of this amazing dish made with love by the women in my family. Traditionally cou cou is made on the stovetop and can be quite tedious and time-consuming. This is my baked version.

COU COU
Prep time: 20 mins. Cooking time: 35 mins
- 2 cups fine cornmeal
- 2½ cups water
- 3 cups okra water

OKRA WATER (FOR COU COU)
Prep time: 10 mins. Cooking time: 10 mins
- 1½ cups okra, finely sliced
- 4 sprigs of fresh thyme or 1 tsp of dried thyme
- ½ cup largely sliced onion
- ½ tbsp salt
- 4½ cups of water (for boiling okras)

1. Place water, okra, salt, thyme, and onion in a pan. Bring to a boil; let boil for 5 minutes.
2. Once boiled, remove okra, onion, and thyme from the water (which now has a slimy consistency). Throw away the thyme stems and onion.
3. Preheat oven to 375 degrees Fahrenheit (F). Place cornmeal in a baking pan. Add 1 cup of water and 2 cups of okra water; stir well. Bake for 10 minutes; reduce oven to 350 degrees F. Add ½ cup of water and ½ cup of the okra water, stir well, then mix in the okras. Bake for an additional 20–25 minutes until the cou cou consistency is similar to mashed potatoes and the top is slightly dry. Remove from oven and let cool slightly.
4. Divide into three servings. Serve with gravy and cucumber salad.

SALT COD GRAVY
Prep time: 15 mins. Cooking time: 20 mins

- 1 fillet salt cod
- 2 garlic cloves, thinly sliced
- 1 cup sliced or canned tomatoes
- ½ cup thinly sliced onion
- 1¼ cups water
- ¼ cup roughly chopped fresh herbs (parsley, cilantro, marjoram)
- ½ tbsp brown (spicy) curry powder
- 1 tbsp vegetable oil
- 4 sprigs of fresh thyme or ½ tsp dried thyme

1. Place salt cod in a small pot, cover with water and bring to a boil; let boil for 5 minutes. Remove cod from hot water; let cool, rinse, and break into small pieces.
2. Heat pan over medium low heat. Place oil in the pan, add curry powder, and let cook until fragrant. Add the onion.

Sauté until onion is translucent, add garlic and thyme, stir, then add cod, stir well. Add tomatoes and water, simmer for 10 minutes. Add fresh herbs. Simmer the gravy for 5 more minutes. Remove from heat.

Vegan option: Omit the salt cod and, after adding fresh herbs, add soy sauce to taste.

CUCUMBER SALAD
Prep time: 10 mins

- ½ long English cucumber, thinly sliced
- 1 tbsp finely minced onion
- 1 tbsp roughly chopped parsley
- ½ tbsp olive oil
- 1½ tbsp freshly squeezed lime juice
- Salt and pepper to taste

Mix ingredients together in a large bowl. Chill.

MUDRAS TO ENHANCE MEDITATIONS

BLACK GODDESS GESTURE (KALI MUDRA)

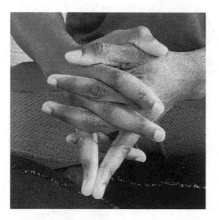

Interlace the fingers, right thumb on top of the left. Straighten the ring fingers and let them touch. Hold for as long as feels comfortable. This mudra helps to clear the mind while grounding and energizing the body.

STABLE AND STEADY GESTURE (STHIRA MUDRA)

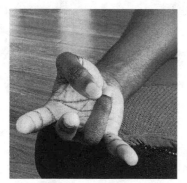 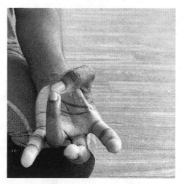

Bring the tip of the right thumb to rest beside the nail of the ring finger on the right hand. Join the tips of the thumb and ring finger on the left hand. Focus on the sensations in your pelvic area and lower back as you practice this mudra. Hold the mudra for 3 to 30 minutes.

MUSIC IDEAS

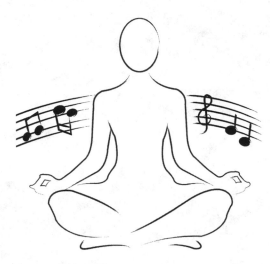

Traditional root chakra music is earthy, tribal, and/or characteristic of your tribe. Root chakra music is ancestral music. Drums are the instruments most associated with root chakra music.

OTHER BALANCING/STRENGTHENING ACTIVITIES

- Earthing, either with the feet directly touching the earth or lying on the earth
- Connecting to nature
- Self-massage for the lower back or dantian (the area below your navel)
- Yoga with active feet
- Massaging the feet
- Mindful walking
- Playing drums, for example the djembe drum
- Submerging oneself in the healthy traditions/practices of one's tribe
- Spending quality time within your tribe/family

Chapter 2

The Sacral Chakra (Svadhisthana) & The Liver Meridian

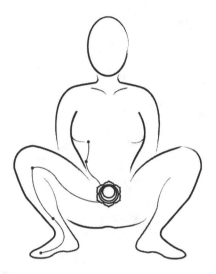

FLOW
ENJOY
PASSION

I move like the live waters.

The sacral chakra, svadhisthana, sits above muladhara approximately 2 inches below our navel, in front of our sacral spine. In Western yoga the sacral chakra governs our body fluids, our reproductive organs, our ability to flow with life, our creativity, and our sensuality. Our sacral chakra is commonly depicted as a six-petaled flower. Unlike muladhara that opens toward the earth, svadhisthana opens toward the front and back of our bodies. Svadhisthana is deeply connected to water. The ways in which we flow in any situation are partially governed by the health of this energy center. The Sanskrit word *svadhisthana* translates to mean 'the residence of the self.' Svadhisthana is located approximately at the same level as our lower dantian. In Traditional Chinese Medicine our dantians are storehouses of vital substances important for good health. Of the three dantians in our bodies, our lower dantian is the most yin.

The liver meridian begins on the top of our feet on the lateral aspect of the big toe. It ascends along the inner leg and wraps around the genitals, then the stomach. Afterwards it enters the gallbladder and liver. The last acupoint on the liver meridian is located in the ribcage in the region under the nipples. From there a deep branch disperses under the ribcage, another branch spreads throughout the lungs, and a third branch ascends, connects to the lips, surrounds the eyes, and terminates at the top of the skull. The liver in Traditional Chinese Medicine holds the office of 'general.' It maintains the correct flow of qi throughout our entire body. It moistens our connective tissues and eyes and regulates our blood and tears. In TCM when qi flows correctly through the body, there can be no pain. We are also emotionally balanced. We acknowledge our emotional states without feeling stifled or overwhelmed by them and we accept our feelings without judgment. We feel our emotions and then return to our natural state—a state of contentment, a state of ever flowing peace.

Healthy flowing energy ensures our bodies are free of emotional and physical pain. A healthy sacral chakra ensures we are gifted with passion. We easily adapt to the ups and downs of life.

Gracefully embracing the tides of our lives helps us to experience the sweetness and beauty that exists in the now. A healthy sacral chakra helps us turn on to the present.

Do you embrace your creativity and sensuality? Can you uplift your energy with thoughts of generosity? Do you honor your passions?

Healthy flowing energy allows us to dance harmoniously with the rhythms of life.

LIFE THEMES

- Expressing one's creativity
- Living with passion
- Flowing easily with the ups and downs of life
- Enjoying and accepting one's innate attractiveness

BALANCED SVADHISTHANA CENTER / HEALTHY LIVER ENERGY	IMBALANCED SVADHISTHANA CENTER / LIVER DYSFUNCTION
A healthy body free of stress-related aches and pains	Hip pain and stiffness
Healthy sensuality	Disorders of the urinary and reproductive organs
Has the ability to easily give birth to ideas and life	Addictions
Expresses emotions in healthy ways	Inability to cope well with emotions
NB: The first point is the only point traditionally associated with liver energy in Traditional Chinese Medicine.	Rigidness
	Frigidity
	Compelled to serve others while neglecting self in most life situations
	NB: The last point is only traditionally found in Western yoga. The remaining points may be associated with other TCM organ systems and chakras.

AFFIRMATIONS

1. I embrace healthy sensuality and pleasure.
2. I enjoy the rhythm of my breath.
3. I accept and delight in my uniqueness.
4. I understand that healthy creativity and passion leads to abundance and joy.
5. I recognize my own innate beauty and enjoy the innate beauty of others.

Making Affirmations Personal

Affirmations are more powerful when they are believable to you. Tailoring affirmations specifically to your unique life situations makes them more believable.

Here is one way to personalize affirmation 3 from the list above—*I accept that my lips are full, broad, and beautiful.*

Here is a personalization of affirmation 4—*I find 30 minutes to paint on weekends because I know this brings me peace.*

YOGA SEQUENCES

GENERAL THEMES

- Practice the yoga sequences in this section with a sense of pleasure to start embodying healthy sacral chakra vitality.
- Congratulate yourself when you catch yourself struggling as you practice. Work on shifting your energy; turn on to something fun/pleasurable/freeing in the pose.
- Breathe into the lower belly, back, hips, and inner groin. Use the breath to create freedom in these areas.
- Do you hold any anger in your body? Anger greatly affects the liver organ and its functioning in Traditional Chinese Medicine. While anger at times can be useful, holding on to anger for long periods of time can affect us (in particular our liver) quite profoundly. Are you ready to release any anger you may be carrying? If you are, feel for the restricted areas where you carry your anger. Can you start to release those restrictions using your breath? Get your breath under those areas as you inhale, and as you exhale feel for releasing any of the sensations associated with your anger. Be aware of any shifts you make with your breath.

Beginners: Breathe in a way that feels good. Breathe into your belly. More advanced beginners: Feel for breathing into your pelvis and groin. It is very helpful to place your hands on these areas as you breathe to help build your awareness of when you are actually getting your breath into these areas. Feel for getting those areas that you are touching to move toward your hands as you inhale. Notice the sensations in that area as you do this.

POSES

Triangle Pose

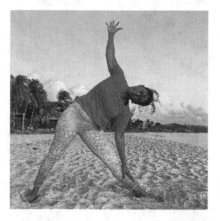

Head to Ankle Preparation

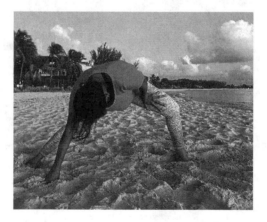

FORREST YOGA SEQUENCE

IDEAS FOR INTENTION

- Can I practice these poses in a way that creates spaciousness and freedom in my hips and pelvis? What feels good/sweet in this pose? Can I focus on that?
- Can I create a sense of playfulness in these poses?

Birthing Squat

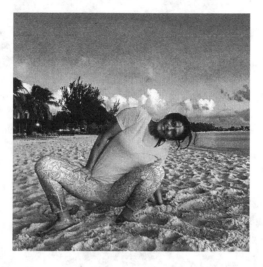

For a longer class, start with: Frog Lifting through Abdominals, Twisting Horse Stance

Pregnant individuals: Abdominal exercises are contraindicated during pregnancy. Ab-less Abdominals with a Mat can be used to replace abdominal exercises. Support your body as needed in the poses. For example, Triangle Pose and Head to Ankle Preparation can be practiced leaning against a wall.

YIN YOGA SEQUENCE AND THE ACUPOINTS

ACUPOINTS

* LR3 (Liver 3) *Great Rushing*

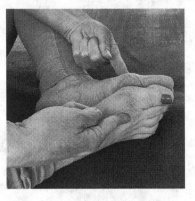

Arguably the most important point along the liver channel, LR3 is frequently used to correct improper qi flow all over the body. It is used clinically to alleviate physical pain, and mental and emotional stress.

Location: In between the metatarsals of the first and second toes, approximately 1 to 1.5 inches from the crease where the first and second toes connect. The spot may be tender.

* SP6 (Spleen 6) *Three Yin Intersection*

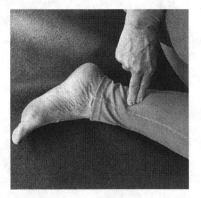

POSES

Seated Butterfly

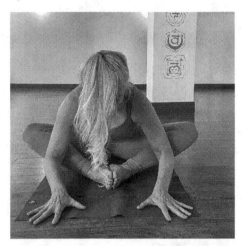

Swan

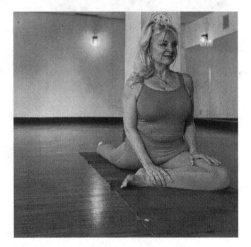

SP6 is the meeting point of the liver, spleen, and kidney channels. As the intersection of three yin meridians, SP6 is an optimal point for increasing yin throughout the body. It is frequently used to treat conditions that affect the liver, spleen, and kidney channels. It nourishes and moves both qi and blood. Blood is the mother of qi and qi is the commander of blood. Healthy movement of both these substances is important for good health. SP6 is commonly used for diseases of the reproductive system and digestive system and for some cases of insomnia. It is contraindicated during pregnancy.

Location: 1 handbreadth directly above K3.

- RN2 (Ren/Conception Vessel 2) *Curved Bone*

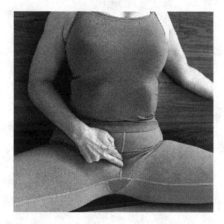

RN2 is located in front of the sacral chakra. Due to its location it is a good point to affect sacral chakra energy.

Location: On the midline of the lower abdomen, feel for the hipbone. RN2 is located immediately above the superior edge of the bone.

Wall Straddle

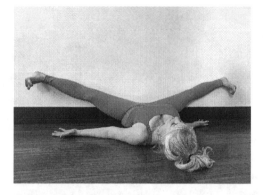

For a longer class, include: Wide Leg Sphinx and Reclining Twist after Swan pose.

Pregnant individuals: Replace Swan with Straddle (side bend variation). Wide Leg Sphinx can be practiced as long as there is no pressure on the belly. Practice Wide Leg Sphinx with a roll or cushions under the thighs, or omit it.

RECIPES

GOGI MANGO SMOOTHIE
Serves 2

In Traditional Chinese Medicine goji berries are frequently used to correct liver dysfunctions. As sour is the taste most associated with the liver in Chinese medicine, lemons and limes are classic food choices for liver dysfunctions such as anxiety and stress. Astragalus root (*Astragalus membranaceus / Astragali radix*) is considered an adaptogen in Western medicine. Adaptogens help the body cope with stress. Mango is a traditional sacral chakra food. Goji berries are commonly used in TCM to support the liver. Be sure to check with your healthcare provider before supplementing with these foods.

- 1 bag astragalus root tea, steeped in 1 cup boiling water (or 1½ cups)
- 1 large ripe mango, peeled and chopped
- ½ tbsp goji berries
- ½ to 1 tbsp freshly squeezed lemon juice
- 1 cup cold water
- 1 tsp honey (optional)

1. Boil water; steep astragalus and goji berries for 5 to 10 minutes. Remove the astragalus and the berries and let the tea cool.
2. Place tea, mango, water, lemon juice, and honey in a blender. Blend until smooth.
3. Pour into two glasses. Top with goji berries.

ORANGE AND PINEAPPLE ATOLE
Serves 2

Citrus fruits help create balance in the sacral chakra and liver meridian. Sour is the taste most associated with the liver in TCM. So even though pineapple is not classified as a citrus fruit, its sour taste means it still can affect the liver meridian and organ. This recipe was inspired by a trip with Mexican friends to the mountains of Xicotepec. Atole is a Mexican hot corn drink that can be made with either fruit or chocolate.

- 1 cup of pineapple chunks (fresh or canned)
- 1 cup of orange juice (freshly squeezed)
- 2½ cups of water
- ⅓ cup of brown sugar
- 1 cinnamon stick
- 6 tbsp masa (nixtamalized corn flour)

1. Place the cinnamon and 1 cup of the water in a small pot. Bring to a simmer over medium heat, then lower the heat.
2. Thoroughly mix 1 cup of the remaining water with the masa; set aside.
3. Blend pineapple chunks with ½ cup of water until smooth. Add to the pot, stir, then stir in the sugar. Cook for approximately 3 minutes.
4. Add the orange juice to the pot, stir, then stir in the masa. Raise the heat to medium and cook until the mixture is simmering and has thickened (no more than 3 minutes).
5. Pour into two mugs. Enjoy!

NB: Feel free to experiment with the sweetness and thickness of the drink by modifying the amounts of sugar and water used.

SALMON TACOS
Serves 6

Communal meals and communal dining are healthy sacral chakra activities. Salmon tacos make a great group meal that allows folks an opportunity to practice creativity.

SWEET POTATO MASH
Prep time: 20 mins. Cooking time: 1 hour

- 2 large sweet potatoes
- 2 pinches of salt (or salt to taste)

1. Heat oven to 425 degrees F. Prick sweet potato with a fork, then cut sweet potato in half lengthways. Roast the potato for 60 minutes.
2. Let potatoes cool. Scoop out the cooked flesh and place it in a bowl; discard the skin and burnt edges.
3. Add salt and mash.

LEMON CREMA
Prep time: 5 mins

- ½ cup sour cream
- 2 pinches salt (or salt to taste)
- ½ tsp lime juice
- 2 tsp favorite pepper sauce (optional)

Place all the ingredients into a small bowl and mix well.

SALSA
Prep time: 10 mins

- 1 large beefsteak tomato, diced
- 1 clove garlic, finely minced
- 1¼ tbsp lime juice
- 3 tbsp freshly chopped cilantro
- Salt to taste

- Cracked black pepper to taste
- 1 tbsp olive oil

Mix tomato, garlic, lime juice, cilantro, and pepper together in a small bowl. Add salt and black pepper as desired.

Vegan option: Omit the salmon and lemon crema and use the bean salsa recipe included.

BEAN SALSA (VEGAN OPTION)

- 1 cup black/kidney precooked beans
- Salsa (see recipe above)

1. Add beans to the salsa mix above.
2. Refrigerate overnight to blend flavors.

SALMON

Prep time: 5 mins. Cooking time: 20 mins

- 2 fillets (approx. 14 ounces each) salmon
- Approx. 1 tsp sea salt (or salt to taste)
- Approx. ½ tsp smoked paprika (or smoked paprika to taste)
- Olive oil

1. Pre-heat oven to 425 degrees F.
2. Line a roasting pan with foil. Spread a bit of olive oil onto the foil to prevent sticking.
3. Place salmon on foil; sprinkle with sea salt and smoked paprika. Drizzle a small amount of olive oil on top, just enough to coat the salmon. Gently rub the salt, paprika, and olive oil into the salmon.
4. Bake for 20 minutes.

TACOS

- 12 hard shell tacos
- Lemon crema
- Salsa
- Salmon
- 6 lettuce leaves, roughly cut

1. Heat taco shells in the oven at 350 degrees F until heated (approx. 3 mins).
2. Place a bit of sweet potato mash, salmon, salsa, lettuce, and lemon crema into each shell. Experiment with quantities and layers. Creating a lettuce wrap instead of a taco is another option.

MUDRAS TO ENHANCE MEDITATIONS

LETTING GO GESTURE (KSHEPANA MUDRA)

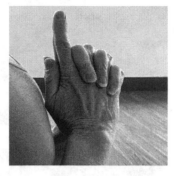

Interlock your fingers, then release your index fingers so they are joined and pointing upward. Hold this position in front of your heart for as long as is comfortable. This mudra gently lifts and circulates qi throughout the body.

FISH GESTURE (MATSYA MUDRA)

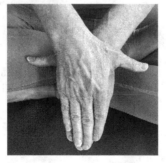

Place the right palm flat over the back of the left hand. The fingers are together and point downward. The thumbs are gently extended away from the index fingers. Focus on the sensations in your pelvis. Hold the mudra for as long as feels comfortable; 5 to 20 minutes is sufficient. Feel free to experiment sometimes, with moving the thumbs in a circular motion while practicing.

MUSIC IDEAS

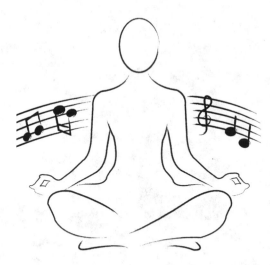

The melodies of sacral chakra music feel sweet and harmonious. Sacral chakra music gently reminds us of the effortless flow of life. The sounds of water, whether it be the ocean or rain, can stimulate and soothe the sacral chakra.

OTHER BALANCING/STRENGTHENING ACTIVITIES

- Socializing with friends and family
- Dancing
- Making music
- Drawing, painting; any activity that allows you to express your creativity
- Qi gong and tai chi
- Singing
- Being close to or on any large body of healthy moving water (may be uncomfortable for folks with trauma associated with water; if you do not feel comfortable around large bodies of water this can be avoided until you feel ready)
- Practicing aparigraha (non-grasping, non-possessiveness)
- Gifting yourself and others with generosity

Chapter 3

The Solar Plexus Chakra (Manipura) & The Spleen and Stomach Meridians

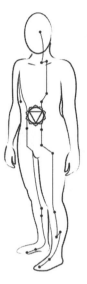

MAKE
POWER
VIGOR

I exercise my power and live to my fullest potential.

Manipura, our solar plexus chakra, is the third major chakra in our energetic anatomy. In Western yoga, manipura is located in front of the spine behind our stomach area and radiates outwards through our middle jiao (middle burner). Our middle jiao in Traditional Chinese Medicine encompasses the area between our navel and our diaphragm. Manipura governs our digestive system, our diaphragm, and our adrenals. When our solar plexus chakra is healthy, we have the energy to live our lives as we truly desire. Our will to achieve is indomitable and we easily assimilate vitality from our environment and our food.

The primary spleen meridian begins in the big toe and ascends along the inner leg to the torso where it connects to the stomach, spleen, and heart. This meridian ends under the armpit in the seventh intercostal space. The primary stomach meridian begins in the face and travels down the throat and torso to connect to the feet, after connecting with the spleen and stomach organs. These two organs and their meridians govern digestion. They ensure the energy from our food enlivens and supports our physical and emotional bodies as well as our mental clarity.

Our self-worth is intricately connected to the health of our solar plexus chakra. Our self-worth is determined by our personal beliefs. Do we choose to believe we all have intrinsic value and unique gifts beneficial to ourselves and humankind? Or do we choose to believe otherwise? Our second brain, also known as our gut feeling, is partially located in this center. Our second brain is another pathway that leads to deeper awareness and truth.

Feed your physical and mental bodies with foods that enliven all of your being.

Nourish your inner fire and acknowledge your self-worth. An inner fire than endures is wisely fueled by our passions, creativity, wisdom, and growth.

Be committed to living with integrity and power!

LIFE THEMES

- Having the physical, emotional, and mental energy to create the life one wants
- A strong sense of self-worth and self-acceptance
- Confidence in one's abilities
- Overcoming over-worry

BALANCED MANIPURA CENTER / HEALTHY STOMACH AND SPLEEN ENERGY	IMBALANCED MANIPURA CENTER / WEAK OR IMBALANCED STOMACH AND SPLEEN ENERGY
Healthy digestive system	Digestive dysfunction, diabetes, energy imbalances, chronic fatigue
Healthy sense of personal power	
Assertive communicator	Body easily bruised
Realistic view of one's abilities and contributions	Has poor discipline
NB: The last three points of both columns are traditionally only found in Western yoga.	An inability to digest new ideas
	An inability to enjoy the richness/sweetness of life
	A tendency to undervalue self and one's contributions
	NB: Discipline in Traditional Chinese Medicine is also connected to other organs.

AFFIRMATIONS

1. My vitality is healthy.
2. I am a lustrous gem; I know my self-worth.
3. Every day I am becoming the best person I can be.
4. I stand up for myself.
5. I recognize my power to be and to achieve.

Making Affirmations Personal

Affirmations are more powerful when they are believable to you. Tailoring affirmations specifically to your unique life situations makes them more believable.

Here is one way to personalize affirmation 1 from the list above—*I have enough energy to walk home from work today. It is a 25-minute walk that I will enjoy.*

Here is a personalization of affirmation 5—*I am able to complete my master's degree in one year.*

YOGA SEQUENCES

GENERAL THEMES

- Visualize your inner city of gems at the solar plexus level as you practice—notice if you can sense what it looks like. Does it look dull or sparkly? Can you use your breath to brighten that area?
- For students who struggle with feelings of unworthiness, feel for the areas of your body that are most affected by that misbelief. Sit tall. Are you ready to breathe fresh energy into those areas?
- Use the energies of both the first chakra (stability, balance) and second chakra (pleasure) to fuel the fire of the third chakra.
- If you worry a lot, notice the thoughts that drive your worry. Can you choose not to engage with those thoughts by changing your focus of attention? Maybe you can ignore worrisome thoughts for 1 breath, 10 breaths, 15 minutes, or the duration of your practice. Focus on your breathing to help you.

Beginners: Fascinate on staying connected to your core/ abdomen with each inhale and exhale.

POSES

Elbow to Knee

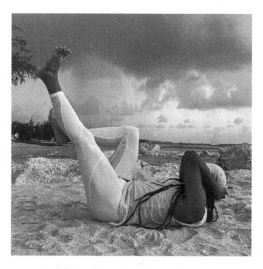

Sun Salutations

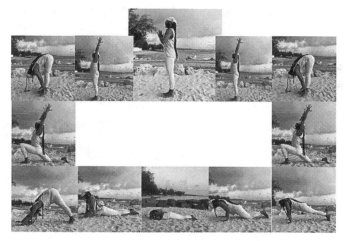

FORREST YOGA SEQUENCE

IDEAS FOR INTENTION

- Turn on your heat. Forrest yoga is normally practiced in a warm environment. Get warm and build up a sweat as you practice.
- Breathe deeply in every pose. Feel your lower ribs expanding with each inhale and releasing as you pull your belly in with each exhale. You can place your hands on your lower ribs to feel if they expand as you inhale.
- Practice this sequence in a way that ignites your inner fire. Can you 'turn on' to the heat?
- As you build heat in the poses, invite and welcome that heat into your cell tissue. Visualize that heat burning away whatever energies you carry in your body that you no longer need.
- Can you practice your yoga in a way that brings self-respect? Some ways you can practice with self-respect include: giving your best effort, breathing deeply, being mindful and respectful of your body's limitations.

Cobra over a Roll

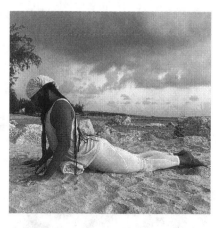

For a longer class, end with: Classical Spinal Twist and/or Reclining Twist

Pregnant individuals: Replace Elbow to Knee with Ab-less Abdominals with a Mat. Replace Cobra over a Roll with Bridge with a Roll between thighs. Practice your Sun Salutations without putting pressure on your belly. Have your legs apart as you move into forward folds. Place a bolster under your thighs when lowering to the floor to perform Cobra so there is no pressure on your belly.

YIN YOGA SEQUENCE AND THE ACUPOINTS

ACUPOINTS

- RN12 (Conception Vessel 12) *Middle Cavity*

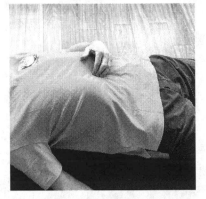

An important point for all digestive disorders, RN12 is also used to improve energy levels in combination with other points. This point is not used during pregnancy.

Location: On the midline of the body, slightly higher than 1 handbreadth above the navel.

- ST25 (Stomach 25) *Heaven's Pivot*

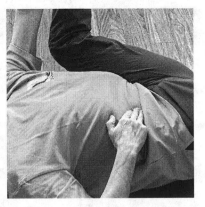

Benefits the intestines and stomach; an important point in the treatment of intestinal disorders. It is not used during pregnancy.

POSES

Half Happy Baby Pose

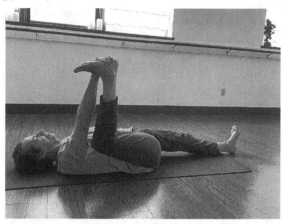

Saddle Pose

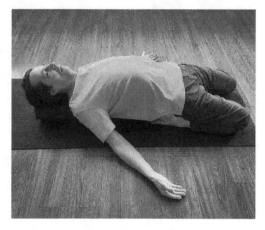

Location: 2 cun (or two thumbs' width) lateral to the navel.

- ST36 (Stomach 36) *Leg Three Miles*

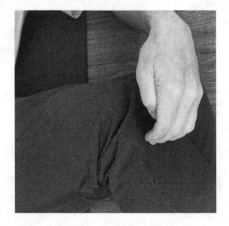

Arguably the most important acupoint of the body, ST36 treats digestive disorders and boosts energy and immunity.

Location: 1 handbreadth below the kneecap on the lateral side of the shin bone.

Reclining Twist

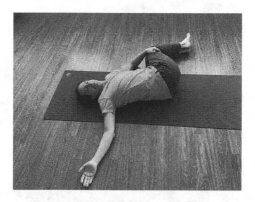

For a longer class, add: Twisting Half Butterfly pose and/or Reclining Deer pose.

Pregnant individuals: As long as there is no pressure on the belly, these poses can be practiced. If lying on your back is uncomfortable, support the back using several pillows or bolsters.

RECIPES

MUM'S APPLE GINGER ELIXIR
Serves 2

All the ingredients in this recipe are known to improve digestion. In TCM, ginger is used to warm the body as well as boost digestion.

- 3 apples (red delicious, gala, fuji, or golden delicious), cored, seeded, and sliced
- 1 cup fresh pineapple chunks
- 4 tsp freshly minced ginger
- 2 tbsp apple cider vinegar

Place pineapple, then apple cider vinegar and apples into a high-speed blender. Add ginger. Blend until smooth. Depending on the type of blender you use, you may need to add a small amount of water. Enjoy!

BANANA TONIC
Serves 2

Ginseng is a timeless gem in TCM. It has been used for several centuries to boost energy and improve digestive function. Bananas make ginseng more palatable. In TCM, bananas have cooling properties. They may be useful for bouts of both constipation and diarrhea. Check with your healthcare provider before supplementing with ginseng.

- 1 Canadian/American ginseng tea bag
- 1½ cups boiling water
- 2 ripe bananas
- ½ tsp brandy essence

- 2 cups almond milk (mylk)
- 2 dashes cinnamon
- Honey to taste

1. Steep ginseng in boiling water for 3 minutes, then remove and discard tea bag.
2. Place bananas, milk, cinnamon, honey, and brandy essence in the blender. Blend until completely smooth.
3. Heat banana mixture in a small saucepan over low heat until warmed through. Add ginseng tea to the pan, stir the mixture. Serve while warm.

CHICKEN BARLEY SOUP
Serves 4

Prep time: 15 mins (for onions, squash, celery, and carrots). Cooking time: 1 hour (dumplings and other ingredients can be prepped during this time)

In TCM a few symptoms associated with a poorly functioning digestive system include heaviness, lethargy, and soft or sticky bowel movements. Barley is a salve for the digestive system and may be able to help with these symptoms. This dish is similar to a typical Barbadian soup. In Barbados, soups are normally quite hearty in consistency. Nourishing, easy-to-digest grains and starchy root vegetables are typical solar plexus chakra foods.

Vegan option: Omit the chicken; use vegetable broth.

- ½ medium-size yellow onion, chopped
- 1 celery stalk, sliced
- 1 medium-size carrot, diced
- 1 butternut squash, peeled, cored, and finely sliced

- 4 chicken thighs, skinned, half the meat removed and chopped into bite-size chunks (marinate the chicken overnight in the juice of half a lime and sufficient water to submerge the chicken)
- ¾ tbsp real salt (or salt to taste)
- 1 tbsp Mrs. Dash Table Blend season mix
- 1 tsp dried thyme
- ½ cup barley
- 2 cups small red potatoes, diced
- ½ tbsp curry
- 2 liters water
- 450 ml bone broth or chicken stock
- 2½ tbsp fresh parsley, chopped
- 2½ tbsp fresh cilantro, chopped
- 1 tbsp vegetable cooking oil

FOR DUMPLINGS

- 1½ cups all-purpose flour or wholewheat flour
- 3 tbsp brown sugar
- Pinch of salt
- ¼ tsp nutmeg
- ½ tsp cinnamon
- ¾ cup hot water

DUMPLINGS

1. Dissolve sugar into hot water; set aside.
2. Combine all the dry ingredients together in a bowl, then add water mix. Mix well with a fork, then knead until the flour has a dough-like consistency.
3. Make 13–14 dumplings; each dumpling should have a diameter of approximately 1½ inches.

SOUP

1. Place a large pot on the stove on medium heat. Add vegetable oil to the pot.
2. Add onions, carrots, celery, and dried thyme to the pot. Sauté until fragrant and bright in color.
3. Add chicken thighs, curry, and Mrs. Dash. Stir. Cover and let cook for 5 minutes.
4. Add squash and barley to the pot. Add salt. Sauté for 1–2 minutes.
5. Add water and bone broth to the pot, bring to a boil, cover, reduce to a rapid simmer, and let cook for 45 minutes. When the soup has simmered for 30 minutes, add the potatoes.
6. Reduce the heat until the soup mixture is slow-simmering. Add dumplings to the pot. Let cook for 5 minutes. Add fresh herbs to the pot. Continue to cook for 5 more minutes.
7. Serve.

MUDRAS TO ENHANCE MEDITATIONS

FIRE GESTURE (AGNI MUDRA)

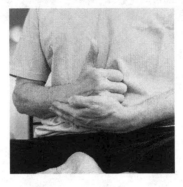

Make a fist with your right hand with the thumb pointing up. Have the palm of the left hand facing upward. Place the fist on top of the palm of the left hand. Hold for as long as is comfortable.

MARK OF SHIVA GESTURE (LINGA MUDRA)

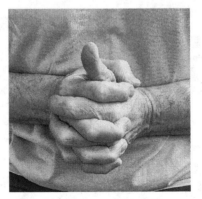

Interlock the fingers with the left thumb on top of the right. Point the right thumb up and encircle it with the thumb and index finger of the left hand. This mudra generates a sense of warmth. It can be held for up to 30 minutes.

MUSIC IDEAS

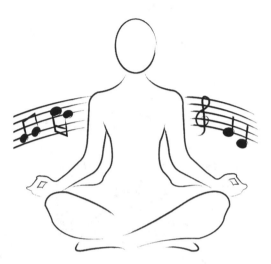

Choose your favorite upbeat songs. Music for your solar plexus chakra makes you want to move and dance.

OTHER BALANCING/STRENGTHENING ACTIVITIES

- Sweat-inducing activities (in moderation)
- Eating daily at the same time
- Uddiyana, agnisara, and nauli (these are intermediate to advanced yogic practices; please learn them from a qualified instructor)
- Pilates
- Abdominal massage (check with a practitioner to ensure this practice is safe for you)
- Consuming easy-to-digest foods at warm (not hot or cold) temperatures
- Intermittent fasting

Chapter 4

The Heart Chakra (Anahata) & The Heart Meridian

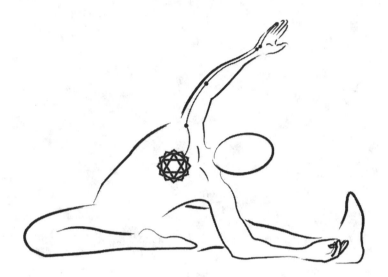

LOVE
KINDNESS
AFFECTION

I am kind to others; I am kind to myself.

Anahata, the heart chakra, is the central chakra of our energetic anatomy. Anahata sits behind the breastbone in the center of our chest. Anahata governs the organs in our chest cavity and upper back. Physically, anahata is level with our body's middle dantian. Dantians in Taoist philosophy are storehouses of our body's vital energies. Our middle dantian is deeply connected to our ability to feel, our emotional awareness, and the vibrancy of our energetic body.

Anahata is love. Its energy opens and diffuses throughout our entire body.

Anahata is the pivot between our lower, more physical energy centers and our upper, more spiritual energy centers. Healthy heart chakra energy raises our vibration to one of wholesome perfection.

In TCM the heart primary meridian begins in the center of our heart and branches out in different directions. The main branch connects to the lungs, then travels down the inner arm to terminate in the little finger. Other branches begin in the heart and connect to the small intestines, the face, and the eyes. In TCM the heart is the 'emperor' of the body. It controls the blood and the blood vessels. It also controls our ability to appropriately relate to friends, colleagues, loved ones, and strangers. Heart health can be seen in our complexion. The heart is affected by all emotions. In Traditional Chinese Medicine the heart is particularly affected by joy.

Touching the heart with the breath is a key component in learning how to connect to our life force. Touching the heart with the breath is integral in learning how to delight in the joy of our spirit.

Reflect on the meaning of anahata. Anahata is defined as an unstruck sound. Is it a sound so pure no mass can make it? Is it a sound that emanates from our nonduality, our true essence?

What words come to mind when you think of love? What qualities symbolize a healthy heart full of love not only for yourself but for others and the world?

May you walk in beauty.

LIFE THEMES

- Being kind to oneself
- Being equally able to give and receive love
- Being able to embody spirit
- Being able to put our heart into the activities we do or pursue

BALANCED ANAHATA CENTER / HEALTHY HEART ENERGY	IMBALANCED ANAHATA CENTER / IMBALANCED HEART ENERGY
Healthy heart and thoracic area	Heart, lungs, breasts, and chest disorders, hypertension, autoimmune disorders
Empathic, nurturing, and compassionate personality	Inability to forgive
Actions motivated by love	Codependent and self-centered personalities
An ability to open to the completeness of life	Inability to self-love
NB: The psychological traits listed in both columns are found only in Western yoga. The last point in this column is also associated with the crown chakra. The thoracic area is also connected to other organs in TCM, notably the lungs.	Apathetic and indifferent individuals
	A tendency to 'perform,' particularly in personal relationships
	NB: Autoimmune disorders are rarely connected to the heart in Traditional Chinese Medicine.

AFFIRMATIONS

1. I honor the desires of my heart.
2. I live in a state of gracefulness and gratitude.
3. Love opens and heals me.
4. I love all that I am.
5. I look within myself for contentment and joy.

Making Affirmations Personal

Affirmations are more powerful when they are believable to you. Tailoring affirmations specifically to your unique life situations makes them more believable.

Here is one way to personalize affirmation 2 from the list above—*I am grateful for the 5 minutes I had today to take a little lunchtime nap.*

Here is a personalization of affirmation 5—*I love that I am learning to better enjoy my own company by spending time dancing alone.*

YOGA SEQUENCES

GENERAL THEMES

- How do you define love? What words would you use to define love? Can you embody the energy of self-love as you practice these routines?
- Can you be kind to yourself as you practice? What does it mean to be kind to myself as I practice?
- Breathe into your heart muscle and/or your heart center. Your heart center is directly behind and slightly below your breastbone. Your heart muscle is beneath your breastbone and slightly to the left of your breastbone in most persons.
- Sometimes love may seem too difficult an emotion to work with. Can you embody a sense of self-respect or self-compassion instead as you practice your postures?
- Feel your hands—they are intimately connected to your heart. You may want to visualize connecting your hands to your heart as you practice.

Beginners: Place your hands over your heart; focus on the sensation of the breath lifting the chest. Imagine fresh oxygenated blood filling the heart with each inhale.

POSES

Seated Side Bend, One Leg Straight with Chest Opener

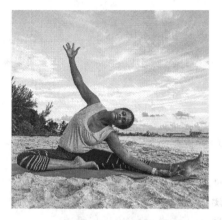

Easy Twisting Warrior

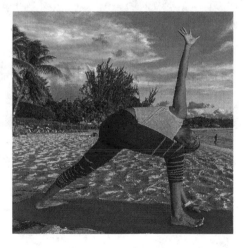

FORREST YOGA SEQUENCE

IDEAS FOR INTENTION

- Can you breathe in a way that caresses your heart or your spirit?
- How does love feel? Can you embody the qualities of love (for example, spaciousness, grace, compassion) in each pose?
- Learn how to embody your spirit in your practice, as an act of love. When we embody spirit we make our body a welcoming home for our spirit. Embodying spirit can feel sparkling or enlivening. Breathe in a way that invites your spirit into all of your body. Start by using your breath to touch your internal landscape (for example, inside your chest) in ways that feel good, inviting, and enlivening.
- Do you struggle as you practice? To struggle is to move away from being kind to oneself. Struggle separates us from the elegance of love. Be able to notice when you move into struggle mode. What happens in your body when you struggle? For example, does your neck and jaw tighten? Do you clench your teeth? Pull back from practicing your poses in those ways.

Camel with a Roll

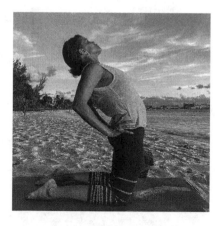

For a longer class, warm up with: Abdominal exercises (for example, Elbow to Knee) and Sun Salutations. Finish with a Reclining Twist.

Pregnant individuals: In Easy Twisting Warrior, have the hand on the floor far away from your front leg so there is no pressure on the belly. Ab-less Abdominals with a Mat can also be added to your sequence.

YIN YOGA SEQUENCE AND THE ACUPOINTS

ACUPOINTS

- RN17 (Conception Vessel 17) *Chest Center*

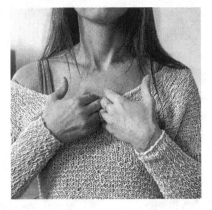

RN17 is the command point of qi. It is deeply connected to the heart chakra because of its location. Its ability to regulate qi in the chest makes it useful for chest and heart pain. It may be used by acupuncturists to improve both breast and lung health.

Location: On the midline of the breastbone, level with the fourth intercostal space, midway between the nipples on men.

- HT8 (Heart 8) *Lesser Palace*

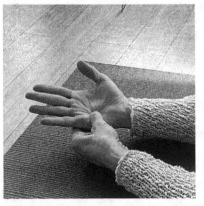

POSES

Reclining Supported Butterfly

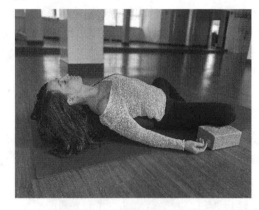

Melting Heart Pose

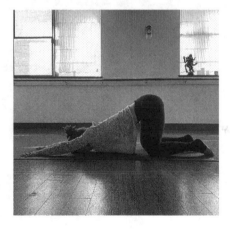

HT8 calms the spirit and clears heat from the heart that may manifest as worry, sadness, palpitations, and chest pain.

Location: Where the tip of the little finger rests when a fist is made.

- HT7 (Heart 7) *Spirit Gate*

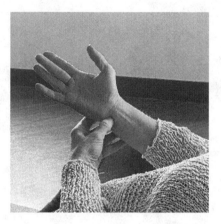

HT7 is commonly used in clinic to relieve emotional agitation and to calm the spirit.

Location: On the wrist crease just proximal to the pisiform bone. Feel for the bone just proximal of the wrist crease, on the palm of the hand.

Sphinx

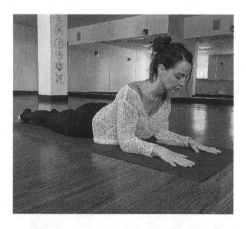

For a longer class, add: Bananasana and/or Reclining Twist.

Pregnant individuals: Practice sphinx with your thighs resting on a bolster or cushions so there is no pressure on the belly. If this is too uncomfortable, replace Sphinx with Supported Bridge. If that too is uncomfortable, omit the pose. Pad your back in Reclining Supported Butterfly with enough pillows or bolsters so the pose is comfortable for you.

RECIPES

GRAPE AND GREEN TEA SMOOTHIE
Serves 2

In TCM, red grapes are recommended for heart deficiencies. In Western medicine, grapes are a good source of potassium, a mineral useful in the regulation of blood pressure. Studies have found green tea can help lower bad cholesterol.

- 1 tea bag of green tea
- 2 cups red seedless grapes
- 2 tsp lemon juice

1. To prepare the green tea, bring hot water to a boil, then let the water cool for 5 minutes. Steep tea bag in 2 cups of hot water for 3 minutes. Remove tea bag. Refrigerate the green tea until almost frozen.
2. Place green tea, lemon juice, and grapes in a blender. Blend until smooth. Enjoy!

STRAWBERRY MOON MILK
Serves 2

Cardamon and turmeric both have cardiovascular benefits. Strawberry moon milk has a lovely pink color. Pink is one of the colors that energizes the heart chakra. In color psychology, pink is associated with compassion, the feminine, and softness. It has a calming effect and is thought to alleviate anger and aggression.

- 1 cup frozen strawberries
- 1 cup hot water
- 2 cups almond milk (mylk)

- Pinch of clove powder
- 2 pinches of turmeric powder
- Pinch of cardamon powder
- 2 pinches of cinnamon powder
- 2½ tbsp brown sugar (or sweetener to taste)

1. Place all the ingredients in a blender. Blend.
2. Place mixture in a pot. Heat on low for 3 to 5 minutes, being careful not to let the mixture boil. Serve while warm.

BLACK RICE SALAD
Serves 4

Salads are commonly associated with the heart chakra. Black rice has a nutty flavor. It contains more protein and fewer carbohydrates than any other type of rice. In ancient China, black rice was known as the forbidden rice because it was reserved exclusively for aristocrats. This nutrient-rich grain is full of antioxidants good for cardiovascular health.

- 1 cup black or brown rice
- 3½ cups water (for cooking rice)
- ½ tsp real salt (or salt to taste)
- ½ tbsp fresh grated ginger
- ½ cup chickpeas
- 2 tbsp chopped scallions
- 2 tbsp cilantro
- 2 tbsp olive oil
- 1 tbsp lime juice
- 1 medium-size beet, roasted and chopped into bite-size chunks
- 1 tbsp mirin or white wine vinegar
- 2 mandarins, peeled and sectioned
- 2 avocados, sliced (optional)

BLACK RICE
Prep time: 5 mins. Cooking time: 35–40 mins

1. Place ½ tsp salt, grated ginger, rice, and water in a pot; bring to a boil.
2. Reduce the heat to a simmer; let the rice cook until all the water evaporates.
3. Turn off the heat. Fluff the rice and let cool.

ROASTED BEETS
Prep time: 2 mins. Cooking time: 1 hour

1. Preheat oven to 400 degrees F. Wash the beets; cut off the leafy tops.
2. Wrap the beets in foil and place in the oven. Cook for approximately 1 hour. Remove from heat and let cool, then chop.

BLACK RICE SALAD
Prep time: 15 mins

1. Place chickpeas, 1 tbsp olive oil, and mirin in a bowl, toss, and set aside. (Do this step preferably before cooking the beets or rice.)
2. Chop scallions and cilantro. Peel and section the mandarins.
3. Mix chickpeas, rice, beets, remaining olive oil, and lime juice in a bowl. Add cilantro, scallions, and mandarins. Toss.
4. Plate the rice in four equal parts. Serve with avocados.

MUDRAS TO ENHANCE MEDITATIONS

LOTUS GESTURE (PADMA MUDRA)

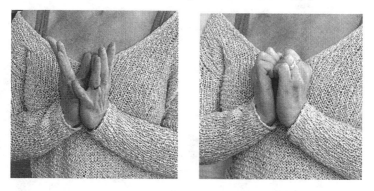

Come into your meditation stance and hold this mudra in front of your heart chakra. Let the base of your palms touch. Allow your fingers to curve in and to touch. Take a few breaths; then, keeping the edges of your little fingers and thumbs touching, stretch your other fingers wide apart. Take 4–5 deep breaths as you hold the mudra, then allow the fingers to touch again. This mudra may be useful in times of grief and loneliness. It helps to rebalance the energy of the heart chakra and opens one to a sense of devotion. You can practice this mudra for up to 30 minutes.

SEAL OF WISDOM GESTURE (JNANA MUDRA)

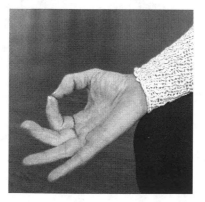

Rest the palms on the lap; join the tips of the thumb and index finger together. The other fingers are relaxed. This mudra helps clear stagnant energy in the chest. It also generates feelings of harmony. This mudra can be held for the duration of your meditation session, as long as the hands are comfortable.

MUSIC IDEAS

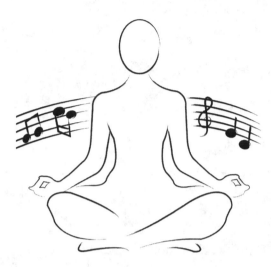

Music for this chakra touches you deeply. Heart chakra music touches your heart and delights you.

OTHER BALANCING/STRENGTHENING ACTIVITIES

- Hugs (for example with people, pets and/or toys)
- Smiling
- Heartfelt touch
- Any activity that delights your heart (that doesn't harm self or others)
- Wearing your happy colors; or wearing pink or green garments
- Enjoying beauty—it could be the beauty of another person, nature, or anything else
- Giving or receiving a hand massage
- Practicing ahimsa (nonviolence), santosha (contentment), and gratitude
- Truthful yet compassionate heartfelt speech

Chapter 5

The Throat Chakra (Vishuddha) & The Lung Meridian

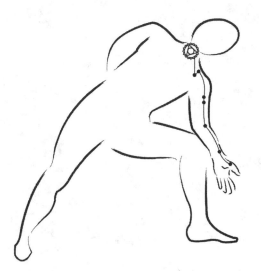

CLEANSE
TRUTH
INTEGRITY

I recognize and I am kind with my truth.

Our fifth chakra, our throat chakra, governs our ability to communicate — within ourselves and with others. The lowest of our higher spiritual centers, our throat chakra sits in front of our cervical vertebra in our throats. In Western yoga it is intricately connected to the glands in our neck, our esophagus, upper back, jaw, our speech, and our voice.

The lung meridian begins in the region of the stomach, descends to connect to the large intestine, ascends to the lungs and the throat, then emerges on the lateral aspect of our chest before it descends along the lateral arm to terminate in our thumbs. In TCM the lung meridian and organ control our breathing and our ability to smell. Our lungs in TCM also affect the health of our skin, body hair, and sweat. Sadness and grief directly affect our lung energy. The lungs also play a major role in immunity and in water regulation throughout the entire body.

The Sanskrit word for our fifth chakra is *vishuddha*, which translates to mean 'purification.' As we evolve into more spiritual beings, we learn to cleanse our bodies of dull untruths that limit our full potential. When our fifth chakra is healthy we walk along our life path with authenticity and integrity. We communicate honestly, speaking our truth while abstaining from gossip. We recognize and regulate the urges of our 'lower' animal self by using our higher spiritual awareness.

Our breath is a healing tool we all possess. The quality of our breathing and air supply affects not only our lung and fifth chakra health but our general mental, emotional, and physical health as well. At any time we can start to cleanse and detox our physical, emotional, and mental bodies by using our breath. Be mindful of holding constrictions in your neck and jaw. These constrictions shut down our fifth chakra and diminish communication between our brain and the wisdom centers of the rest of our body.

Breathe deep, live your life, speak your truth!

LIFE THEMES

- Speaking your truth compassionately
- Listening to and honoring the truth of others, while honoring your own truth
- Cleansing the body and mind of falsehoods and untruths
- Communicating, both verbally and physiologically, in healthy ways

BALANCED VISHUDDHA / HEALTHY LUNG ENERGY	IMBALANCED VISHUDDHA / WEAK LUNG ENERGY
Healthy respiratory system Good immunity Healthy thyroid Healthy neck Expresses oneself easily, expresses oneself truthfully with grace NB: *The first two points in both columns are the only two points commonly connected to lung energy in Traditional Chinese Medicine. Throat disorders are also commonly connected to lung energy but not always.*	Weak immunity Weak voice Beliefs that we cannot express our needs, or truth, in kind ways; gossiping, loudness, stuttering Throat, thyroid, parathyroid disorders Chronic neck stiffness, jaw pain

AFFIRMATIONS

1. I speak kindly to myself and to others.
2. What I have to say is worthy of being listened to. My voice is strong and compelling.
3. I delight in healthy self-expression.
4. I regularly purify my body and thoughts.
5. I breathe slowly and deeply.

Making Affirmations Personal

Affirmations are more powerful when they are believable to you. Tailoring affirmations specifically to your unique life situations makes them more believable.

Here is one way to personalize affirmation 2 from the list above—*My kids listen to what I have to say when I speak calmly to them.*

Here is a personalization of affirmation 4—*I spend 20 minutes weekly in the sauna near my office.*

YOGA SEQUENCES

GENERAL THEMES

- Practice the poses in this section in a way that feels freeing or cleansing to your physical, emotional, and mental bodies.
- Feel the sensations in your neck, jaw, and shoulders in each pose.
- Do you carry sadness, grief, or guilt in your body? Grief and sadness deeply affect the lungs in Traditional Chinese Medicine. Where do you carry these emotions? For example, grief is commonly felt in the chest and in and around the heart. Can you use your breath to bring healing energy to these areas?
- Are you being truthful about your body's abilities as you practice? (Your body's capability to perform specific movements may change daily.) Are you honoring your abilities as you practice, while still allowing some room for growth and challenge?

Beginners: Work on fully relaxing the neck and jaw in all your postures.

POSES

Seated Side Bend, One Leg Straight with Neck Release

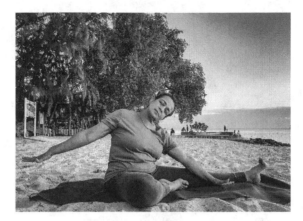

Extended Warrior Variation

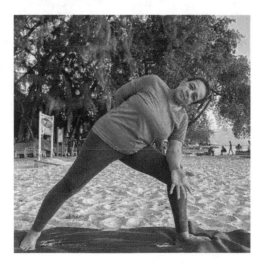

FORREST YOGA SEQUENCE

IDEAS FOR INTENTION

- Turn the heat up; get a cleansing sweat going. Forrest yoga is normally practiced in a heated room.
- Focus on keeping your jaw and neck relaxed as you practice each posture and transition from posture to posture. Take a few lion's breaths while in your poses to help release tension from your jaw, neck, and mouth.
- Can you be expressive in your yoga poses? What attitude/ quality do you most want to express in your asana today? For example, gratitude, balance, self-love, strength—you choose.
- Can you use each breath as a tool to cleanse your inner landscape? If you can't feel this, can you visualize or imagine it happening with each breath you take?

Forward Fold with Neck Traction

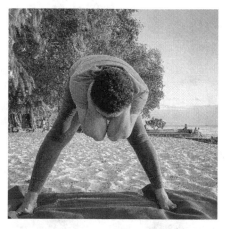

For a longer class, begin with: Elbow to Knee and Sun Salutations

Pregnant individuals: Replace Elbow to Knee with Ab-less Abdominals with a Roll. Extended Warrior Variation can be practiced against a wall.

YIN YOGA SEQUENCE AND THE ACUPOINTS

ACUPOINTS

- G20 (Gall Bladder 20) *Wind Pool*

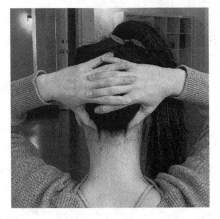

G20 is commonly used to create mental clarity. It is also commonly used to release tension from the back of the neck and skull.

Location: Clasp hands behind the back of the skull. The thumbs should naturally fall into depressions below the skull. These depressions are the approximate location of G20.

- LU1 (Lung 1) *Middle Palace*

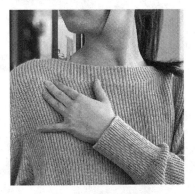

POSES

Seated Neck Release

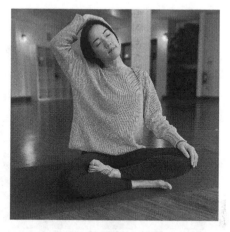

Bananasana

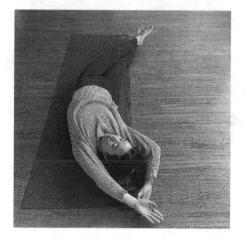

LU1 is commonly used in clinic to stop coughs and improve breathing.

Location: In a depression created on the lateral chest when the hand is extended in front of the body.

- LU9 (Lung 9) *Supreme Abyss*

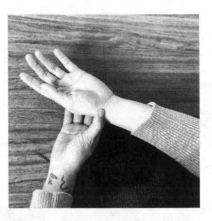

LU9 is an important point on the lung channel to strengthen the lungs and lung functions.

Location: At the lateral edge of the wrist crease. First locate HT7 (see heart chakra points). LU9 is level with HT7 to the outside of the radial pulse felt at the wrist.

Seated Spinal Twist

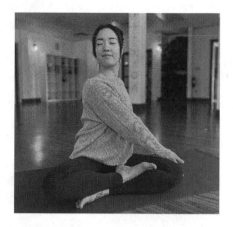

For a longer class, add: Sphinx, Straddle (side bend variation).

Pregnant individuals: Replace Sphinx with Supported Bridge, or practice Sphinx with the thighs over cushions or a bolster, so there is no pressure on the belly.

RECIPES

LEMON CHAI PUDDING
Serves 2

Lemons in TCM are sometimes used to relieve coughs and reduce phlegm in the lungs. Yogurts help moisten the lungs.

- ¼ cup white chai seeds
- ¾ cup water
- 1 cup vanilla-flavored or coconut yogurt
- 2–3 tbsp honey
- ¾ cup coconut milk
- 3–4 tbsp freshly squeezed lemon juice
- Optional toppings: for example blueberries or raspberries

1. Place chai seeds and water in a small container. Cover; let sit overnight in the refrigerator.
2. Mix all the ingredients. Divide into two servings.
3. Top with your favorite berries/seeds/nuts.

CINNAMON PEAR CIDER
Serves 2

Chinese pears are commonly used in Traditional Chinese Medicine to soothe a dry cough. Cinnamon is also frequently used in Traditional Chinese Medicine to ward off respiratory infections that present with chills, no sweating and achiness.

- 2 Chinese pears
- 2 cups water
- 2 gala apples (or any other sweet apple)
- Honey or maple syrup to taste

1. Core and peel the pears and apples.
2. Blend the fruits with water in a high-speed blender until smooth.
3. Place blended pear and apple mixture in a small pot. Bring to a low simmer. Simmer for 5 minutes. Remove from heat.
4. Add sweetener to taste. Serve hot.

SINGAPORE NOODLES
Serves 2–3

Singapore noodles are believed to be originally from Hong Kong. This dish is flooded with herbs and spices which—when used appropriately in TCM—boost lung function. Some acrid foods when used in moderation support lung health. In TCM, mushrooms boost lung qi and help clear heat and phlegm from the lungs.

- 110g rice vermicelli
- 1 liter water
- 2 tsp sesame seed oil
- 2 tbsp grapeseed oil or vegetable oil
- 1 tbsp curry powder
- 1 tbsp Bragg's liquid aminos or soy sauce
- ½ tsp sugar
- 2 garlic cloves
- 1 tsp freshly grated ginger
- ½ bell pepper, sliced
- ⅓ cup chopped yellow onion
- ¾ cup vegetable broth
- 1 cup mung bean sprouts
- ½ cup chopped parsley
- 1 medium carrot, julienned
- 1 cup chopped mushrooms

- Sea salt to taste
- Avocado, sliced

Prep time: 20 mins. Cooking time: 20 mins

1. Heat grapeseed oil on low heat; add curry and cook until fragrant. Remove from heat.

2. Bring 1 liter of water to boil. Place noodles in a large bowl, pour boiling water over noodles, and soak for approximately 5 minutes. Drain noodles, place on a cutting board, and cut in quarters. Return noodles to the bowl; add curry mixture, aminos, and sugar. Toss well.

3. Heat 1 tsp sesame seed oil on medium heat in a nonstick pan. Add ginger and onion, sauté until fragrant; add bean sprouts, cook for 2 minutes. Add salt to taste, then bell pepper. Continue cooking until veggies are tender-crisp. Transfer to a bowl.

4. Return pan to the heat. Heat the remaining sesame seed oil; add mushrooms and garlic, season with salt to taste. Cook mushrooms until they sweat. Add carrots; continue to cook until carrots are tender-crisp. Transfer to a bowl.

5. Return pan to the heat. Add broth to the pan and bring to a simmer. Add noodles and cook, stirring frequently until liquid is absorbed. Turn off the heat. Add vegetables; toss to combine. Mix in parsley and lime juice. Serve immediately with sliced avocados.

MUDRAS TO ENHANCE MEDITATIONS

PURIFIED GESTURE (VISHUDDHA MUDRA)

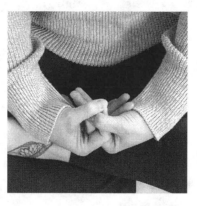

Loosely interlock the fingers; the tips of the index fingers touch the tips of the thumbs. Relax your shoulders and focus on the sensations in the throat and jaw. This gesture strengthens and balances the throat and helps enable authentic communication. This mudra can be held for anywhere from 5 to 30 minutes.

SILENCE OF THE VOID GESTURE (SHUNYA MUDRA)

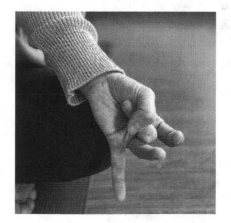

Have your palms resting on your thighs, facing up. Flex your middle fingers toward the base of your thumbs. Bend your thumbs over the middle fingers while keeping the other fingers relaxed and extended. This mudra may be useful in the alleviation of throat disorders connected to the ears, and ear disorders such as tinnitus and reduced hearing. This mudra is a sedating mudra. It should not be practiced for long periods of time if the throat and ears are healthy. Five minutes of practice is sufficient.

MUSIC IDEAS

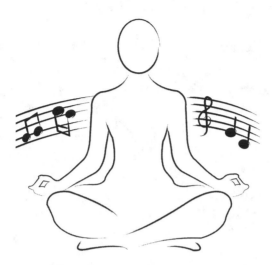

Music that makes you sing with gusto! Music or chants that create a sense of clarity in your brain, throat, and lungs.

OTHER BALANCING/STRENGTHENING ACTIVITIES

- Figure 8 movements with your jaw
- Public speaking (in moderation)
- Breath control (pranayama) exercises
- Journaling
- Lion's breaths
- Authentic communication, with self and with others
- Gargling with warm saltwater (should be done no more than 2–3 times daily)
- Healthy air supply

Chapter 6

The Brow Chakra (Ajna) & The Gallbladder and Governing Meridians

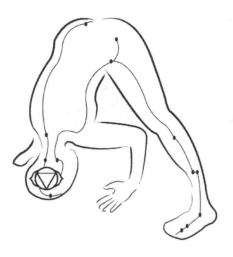

CLARITY
SIGHT
WISDOM

Submerged in the stillness, my vision is clear.

Our sixth chakra, ajna, commonly referred to as the third eye, is our center of intuitive and physical sight. The Sanskrit word *ajna* translates to mean 'center of perception,' as well as 'center of command.' Ajna sits at the top of our spinal column in the space between our midbrow area and the base of our skull. It governs our brain, our face, our neurological system, our sinuses, and our eyes. It is through ajna that we are able to perceive our reality—ourselves, the people around us, our world—and command our existence.

Of the meridians that can affect visual and mental clarity, the gallbladder and governing vessel meridians are quite analogous to the sixth chakra. The gallbladder meridian begins at the outer eye, travels over the lateral skull and lateral aspect of the body, to end at the fourth toe. The governing vessel begins in the lower abdomen, descends to the perineum, then ascends via the interior of the spinal column to the brain, where it terminates at the upper lip. Several acupoints along the gallbladder meridian are used clinically for visual disturbances and mental clarity. Several acupoints along the governing vessel are also used to boost mental clarity and improve vision. The gallbladder is very closely connected to the liver. Some gallbladder acupoints are frequently used to support liver function. The effectiveness of the liver to some extent is dependent on the health of the gallbladder. The liver in TCM is responsible for the smooth flow of qi. It also affects our ability to see.

The gallbladder in TCM is known as the rectifier, and the issuer of decisions. Healthy gallbladder energy gives us the courage to make morally balanced decisions.

Our physical and intuitive vision help us to perceive the truths of our lives. Our ability to create our future is dependent on sound and clear judgment.

What actions can you take to ensure that your vision is clear and focused?

How do you consciously shape and create your future?

LIFE THEMES

- Perceiving the duality of life
- Seeing all life deeply, not only on superficial levels
- Recognizing your truths and needs, as well as the truths and needs of others
- Trusting one's inner knowledge

BALANCED AJNA	IMBALANCED AJNA
Healthy vision	Eye and pituitary gland disorders, poor vision, headaches
An ability to accurately perceive the world	
Can easily visualize things/ outcomes	Logic-focused, intellectually arrogant
Mentally, emotionally, and spiritually intelligent	Perception issues
	Difficulties strategizing
Intuitive—trusting of one's instincts	Self-identity challenges
Decisive	NB: The gallbladder and governing meridians can be used to treat eye disorders, even when the dysfunction is caused by problems with another TCM organ or by an external pathogen.

AFFIRMATIONS

1. I see with clarity.
2. I perceive with equanimity the truths of my life.
3. I trust my inner voice.
4. I make time for silence and introspection.
5. I delight in my imagination, and I understand its power to create my reality.

Making Affirmations Personal

Affirmations are more powerful when they are believable to you. Tailoring affirmations specifically to your unique life situations makes them more believable.

Here is one way to personalize affirmation 2 from the list above—*I am primarily judged by my actions.*

Here is a personalization of affirmation 5—*I can see with my mind the home I think is absolutely best for my family.*

YOGA SEQUENCES

GENERAL THEMES

- During your practice, focus on the feeling of your body as you move through the different postures. Feel your chest, your neck, your ankles, your lower back, your arms, all your body. Use feeling to increase your awareness of—or ability to see—your body.

- Visualization can be a useful tool in healing. Do you believe you create your reality? What qualities do you want more of in your present life? For example, more energy, more pleasure, more joy. Can you work on embodying those feelings as you practice your yoga?

- If you have an injured area, can you breathe into it? Can you feel your breath moving into that area? Or can you visualize each inhale entering that area, bringing healing energy to it? It is helpful to place your hands on the area you are trying to bring breath to. As you inhale, feel your area expanding into your hands. Notice the sensations in your area as you do this.

- Do you frequently feel anxious or nervous? Where in your body do you carry these emotions? For example, do you carry nervousness in your abdomen? Can you start to breathe into these areas?

- Breathe into your brain. This may feel like a brightening or expansion in the skull. If this is difficult to feel, visualize each breath filling the skull and brain.

- Embrace silence in your practice. You can start to do this by focusing your attention on the sensations of your body in each pose. Embracing silence also requires not conversing or engaging with thoughts as they enter your awareness.

POSES

Bridge

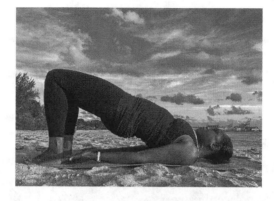

Dolphin

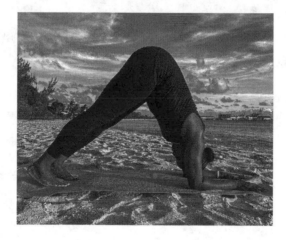

Beginners: Work with your eyes closed in some or all of the postures. This helps develop proprioception.

NB: Practicing yoga with the eyes closed can be useful when suffering from a headache.

FORREST YOGA SEQUENCE

IDEAS FOR INTENTION

- Choose a spot, for example your upper back or brain, that you would like to bring more breath to; breathe into that area in each pose. Fascinate on that area—can you start to notice the size, shape, density, and texture of that area? Does the area change when you direct your inhales into it?
- Are you aware of a belief you have about yourself or others that negatively affects your reality? Where in your body do you carry that belief? Can you breathe into that area as you practice, to see if you can create change in that area using your breath?
- Learn to watch your thoughts without engaging with them. Move into what is known as 'the second attention,' a deeper level of awareness that exists under the chatter of the brain.

Downward-Facing Dog

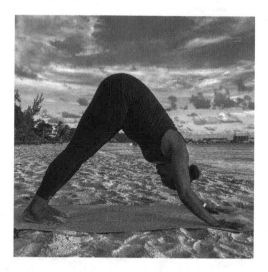

For a longer class, start with: Elbow to Knee, then Sun Salutations after Bridge.

Pregnant individuals: Replace Elbow to Knee with Ab-less Abdominals with a Mat.

YIN YOGA SEQUENCE AND THE ACUPOINTS

ACUPOINTS

- YINTANG (*Hall of Impression*)

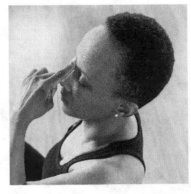

Yintang is an extra point. Extra points do not belong to any of the 14 major meridians. Yintang helps calm the mind and is useful for sinus and vision problems. It may also aid in the treatment of insomnia, anxiety, and agitation.

Location: At the midpoint between the eyebrows.

- GB1 (Gallbladder 1) *Pupil Crevice*

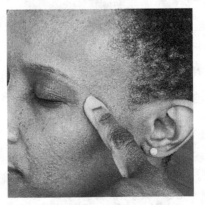

POSES

Child's Pose

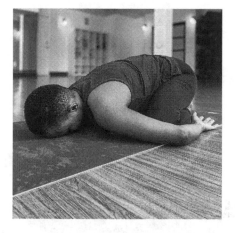

Fire-Breathing Dragon Variation

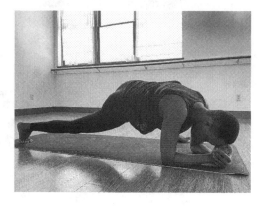

GB1 is used commonly for eye disorders. It is also used for temporal headaches and dizziness.

Location: In a depression just lateral to the outer canthus of the eye.

- DU20 (Governing Vessel 20) *Hundred Meetings*

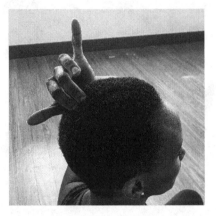

DU20 assists in the creation of mental clarity and helps soothe mental agitation. It may be useful in the treatment of dizziness, heaviness, or dullness that affects thinking.

Location: Place the heels of the hand on the anterior and posterior hairlines and extend the middle fingers toward each other. DU20 is located approximately 1 inch anterior to where the middle fingers touch.

Caterpillar Variation

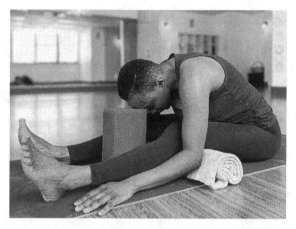

For a longer class, add scalp and eye massage—using the fingertips, press into the scalp and move the fingertips in slow circular motions. Massage around the eye sockets, not onto the eyes. The massage should feel good. Pay particular attention to any sensitive spots and the acupoints mentioned.

Pregnant individuals: Practice Child's Pose and Caterpillar with the legs open at least hip distance apart, so there is no pressure on the belly.

RECIPES

CHOCOLATE LAVENDER SHAKE
Serves 2

Lavender is commonly used in the West to calm the senses. Research has also found blackberry supplementation may be useful at protecting the brain from age-related diseases.

- 80g white vegan chocolate (your favorite white chocolate bar)
- 2 cups homemade almond milk
- 2 tsp lavender officinalis buds
- ½ cup boiling water
- Blackberries to garnish

1. Steep lavender buds in boiling water for 10 minutes; strain.
2. Pour lavender tea and almond milk into a bowl. Place in the freezer; chill.
3. Place milk and lavender mixture, and white chocolate in a blender. Blend until smooth.
4. Pour into two glasses. Top with blackberries.

ROSEMARY VEGAN CHOCOLATE
Serves 2

Compounds in rosemary may have the ability to improve memory and prevent neurological brain damage. Rosemary may also be useful in protecting the eyes from macular degeneration. Dark chocolate is a quintessential third eye chakra food. Flavanols found in dark chocolate may benefit brain function.

- 3 cups homemade almond milk (or pure almond mylk unsweetened) *NB: The milk should be thick and creamy*
- 10g of your favorite dark chocolate bar
- Pinch of salt
- 2 tbsp brown sugar (or to taste)
- 2 tsp dried rosemary leaves

1. Place chocolate in a small pan.
2. Place the pan on the lowest heat. Add salt and rosemary.
3. Move the chocolate around until it is melted; be careful not to burn.
4. Whisk in the milk and sugar. Heat until bubbles are barely rising to the top of the mix.
5. Remove from the heat, strain, and enjoy!

NUTTY TOFU WRAP
Serves 2

- 1½ cups baby spinach
- 4 large lettuce leaves (iceberg or butter lettuce)
- 1 pack firm tofu
- 1 tbsp sesame seed oil
- ½ cup almond or peanut butter
- 2 tbsp Bragg's liquid aminos or your favorite soy sauce
- ½ tbsp of your favorite pepper sauce
- Half a small red onion, thinly sliced
- ½ cup hot water
- ½ cup snow peas
- 1 avocado, cut into bite-size pieces
- 2 tbsp cilantro
- Salt to taste
- ¼ tsp garlic powder
- Olive oil
- Lemon

1. Cut tofu into bite-size pieces; toss well with olive oil. Grill in the oven, flip tofu over, and grill until all edges of the tofu are toasted light brown. Remove from heat.

2. In a small pan heat ½ tbsp sesame seed oil. Add snow peas, stir; add garlic powder, and salt to taste. Sauté for 1 minute. Add 1 tbsp of water to snow peas. Cook until water is completely absorbed and the snow peas are bright green in color. Remove from heat.

3. In a separate pan mix the nut butter, hot water, and soy sauce thoroughly. Heat until the mixture starts to simmer, add the tofu pieces. Immediately remove from heat.

4. Place the spinach, snow peas, tofu, avocado, and onions onto the lettuce leaves. Lightly drizzle with lemon juice and olive oil. Serve with cilantro sprinkled on top.

MUDRAS TO ENHANCE MEDITATIONS

OBSTACLE-REMOVING GESTURE (GANESHA MUDRA)

Your right palm faces up while your left palm faces down. Bend your fingers and hook them together. Your hands may be in front of your navel or resting on your lap. Hold for as long as feels comfortable. This gesture gently opens and lifts the upper chest. It promotes confidence and determination. It is also a useful gesture to strengthen solar plexus chakra energies.

PRAYER GESTURE (NAMASKAR MUDRA)

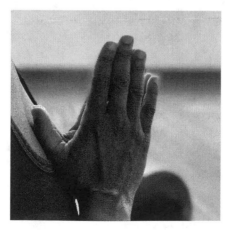

Bring your hands into prayer position in front of the heart. Hold for as long as is comfortable. This mudra reduces stress and calms the mind. It is also a useful mudra for the heart organ and meridian and the crown chakra.

MUSIC IDEAS

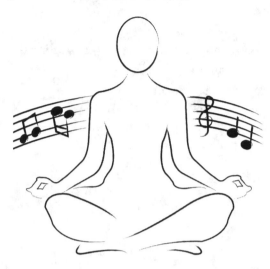

Choose calming, meditative music; binaural beats; soothing flute music.

OTHER BALANCING/STRENGTHENING ACTIVITIES

- Eye exercises
- Dream journaling and dream interpretation
- Listening to and honoring your 'gut feelings'
- Practicing trataka (gazing exercise)
- All forms of meditation
- Activities that strengthen proprioception
- Engaging in svadhyana (self-study)

Chapter 7

The Crown Chakra (Sahasrara) & The Governing and Conception Meridians

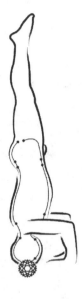

DIVINE
SACRED
GRACE

In the present, I am free.

Sahasrara chakra, our thousand-petaled lotus, sits just on top of our head. Sahasrara connects us to our divinity and governs our cerebrum or higher brain. It nourishes our spirituality and gifts us with heavenly grace. It filters down through all of our being and allows divine wisdom a voice in all aspects of our lives.

The governing vessel (Du) begins in the lower abdomen, ascends along the spine, traverses over the top of the skull, then connects with the conception vessel (Ren). The conception vessel also begins in the lower abdomen. Its main branch ascends along the front of the body where it connects with the governing vessel in the area of the mouth. The conception and governing vessels are considered inseparable, like night and day. Together these extraordinary meridians fuel our body's principal yin and yang. They can be used to treat conditions that affect any of the organs of the body.

Both meridians have branches that travel beside each other. Both originate from the same source, the lower dantian, and travel upward through the body, connecting to our middle and upper dantians. The dantians store the vital substances necessary for life. Imagine them as reservoirs in the body, while the meridians can be compared to rivers. The lower dantian is associated with our essence. Our essence determines our physical development, our vitality, and our life span. The middle dantian stores the fundamental qi that nourishes and supports our entire body. It is deeply connected to our heart, our lungs, and our emotions. Our upper dantian houses the purest of our vital substances—our spirit. Our spirit enables us to think. It facilitates spiritual awareness and growth, and guides our intentions, our life purpose. Together, our Du and Ren create the microcosmic orbit commonly used in qigong to cultivate energy and consciousness.

We understand our life's purpose through the energies of our seventh chakra and upper dantian. The wisdom of our upper dantian spreads throughout our body via our meridians.

Work to recognize and develop your unique gifts through kind thoughts, kind actions, and faith. Ask yourself: What positive actions can I take to create inner balance and peace? As our ability to live fully in the present increases, so too does our capacity for grace.

Namaste.

LIFE THEMES

- Finding inner peace and/or inner satisfaction
- Recognizing the beauty and oneness of all beings
- Recognizing the divinity in all beings
- Living in a way that nurtures what is sacred

BALANCED SAHASRARA CENTER	IMBALANCED SAHASRARA CENTER
Lives frequently in a state of inner peace and satisfaction	Mania-depression, panic attacks
Understands one's purpose	Lacking purpose
Recognizes and honors the spiritual truths of all religions	An inability to recognize common truths in all religions
Empathetic	Apathetic
NB: The last point of each column is also associated with the heart chakra.	NB: The first point is also associated with the sacral and heart chakras.

AFFIRMATIONS

1. I am deserving of unconditional grace.
2. I honor both my physical and spiritual needs.
3. I make time for the sacred in my life.
4. I am present.
5. There is beauty all around me.

Making Affirmations Personal

Affirmations are more powerful when they are believable to you. Tailoring affirmations specifically to your unique life situations makes them more believable.

Here is one way to personalize affirmation 3 from the list above — *I pray before each meal.*

Here is a personalization of affirmation 4 — *I am present as I read this book.*

YOGA SEQUENCES

GENERAL THEMES

- Practice staying present in your yoga practice. Thoughts (regarding your past and your present) will naturally come to mind as you perform the poses. Focus on the sensations in your body as you practice, as a way of staying present. Can you bring your best quality of attention, your best effort, into your practice? Whatever that may be for the day?
- Focus on feeling every inhale and exhale as a gift—a gift of aliveness; a blessing.
- Choose a word that symbolizes an aspect of your divinity; for example, grace, serenity, humility. Can you use your breath in a way that helps you embody the qualities of that word? Please note that attempting to embrace qualities you are not quite ready for may result in failure and disappointment. Choose a word or sensation you can work with.
- Each yoga posture has its own energy. Can you nurture yourself with the energy that each pose provides? Notice what feels good about a pose, focus on that energy, consume it as you inhale; use it to nourish your body, mind, and soul.
- Practice feeling the lower six chakra regions of your body in your practice as a way of being present.

Beginners: Focus solely on each inhale and exhale. Try not to engage with or respond to thoughts as they come into your awareness.

POSES

Half Moon

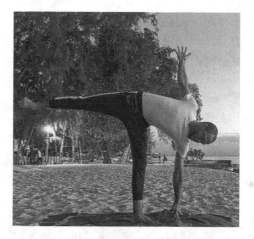

Headstand

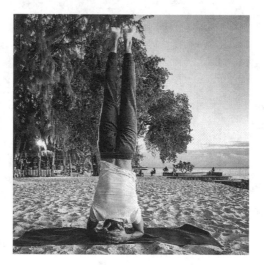

FORREST YOGA SEQUENCE

IDEAS FOR INTENTION

- Get present. (See general themes in this chapter.)
- Learn to embody spirit. Learning to embody spirit means figuring out how to move and breathe in a way that enlivens your internal landscape, so it is a home for your spiritual body. Notice how it feels to take a deep breath into your lungs and your abdomen. When we embody spirit, our breath brightens and expands our internal world. Our breath feels very good; it feels enlivening.
- Each pose has its own energy. The energy you feel in Warrior 1, for example, is different from the energy you feel in Dolphin. Can you feed (nourish) yourself with the different energies the poses provide?
- Breathe through all the lower chakras as a way of becoming present. Throughout your poses, use your breath to connect to all of your energy centers in a 'beauty way.' To do this, perhaps you may want to visualize the different colors of the chakras filling your body as you breathe and move. Perhaps you may want to focus on feeling an opening or brightening in the different energy centers as you breathe and move.

Shoulderstand

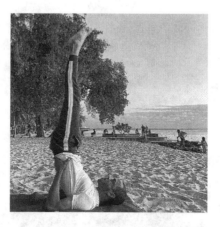

For a longer class, add: Elbow to Knee and Bakasana

Pregnant individuals: Support your body with props as necessary. In Half Moon the supporting hand can rest on blocks. Shoulderstand can be practiced with the feet resting on a wall. Stay very alert to how you feel when coming into, staying in, and getting out of these postures. It is advised that you do not practice these inversions if these postures were not in your practice prior to your pregnancy. If you would still like to practice them, please do so with the assistance of a qualified instructor.

YIN YOGA SEQUENCE AND THE ACUPOINTS

ACUPOINTS

- DU26 (Governing Vessel 26) *Man's Middle*

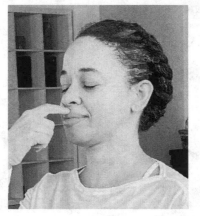

This point revives consciousness and is used to re-establish yin-yang harmony.

Location: Midway between the tip of the nose and the edge of the upper lip on the midline of the face.

- LR3 (Liver 3) *Great Rushing*

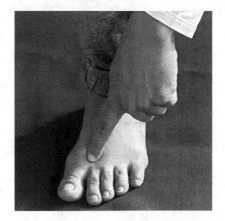

POSES

Toe Squat

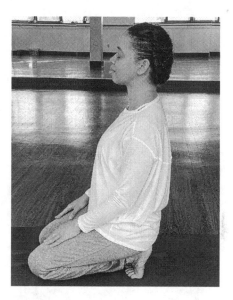

Dragon Flying High

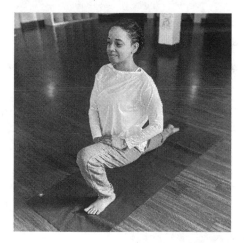

LR3 corrects improper qi flow throughout the body. When qi flows correctly we are emotionally balanced, and closer to our natural state of being. In our natural state we are more receptive to the present and consequently to our divine nature.

Location: In between the metatarsals of the first and second toes, approximately 1 to 1.5 inches from the crease where the first and second toes connect. The spot may be tender.

- RN14 (Conception Vessel 14) *Great Gateway*

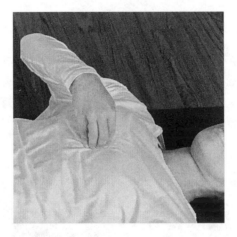

RN14 regulates the heart and chest and can be used for emotional distress, anger, and disorientation.

Location: RN14 is located approximately 2 handbreadths above the umbilicus. Massage gently as it may be very tender. Tapping RN14 before resting in savasana may help you relax.

Savasana

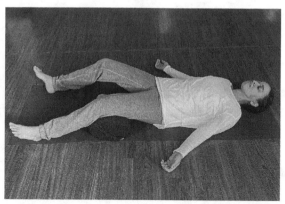

For a longer class, add scalp massage—using the fingertips, press into the scalp and move the fingertips in slow circular motions. The massage should feel good. Pay particular attention to any sensitive spots.

Pregnant individuals: Rest in savasana with the back elevated by cushions or bolsters so the pose is comfortable. Practice Dragon so there is no pressure on the belly.

RECIPES

LEMON BALM ICED TEA
Serves 2

Lemon balm soothes the symptoms of stress and may help improve cognitive function. It should not be used continuously. Check with your healthcare professional before using this herb.

- 2 lemon balm tea bags
- 2 cups of hot water
- Freshly squeezed juice of two grapefruits
- 2 cups of ice
- Honey or favorite sweetener to taste

1. Steep tea bags in hot water for 10 minutes. Remove tea bags and let the tea cool.
2. Add tea, ice, grapefruit juice, and honey to blender. Blend.
3. Serve immediately.

GOTU KOLA GINGER TEA
Serves 2

Ginger is a superfood commonly used for indigestion and nausea. Ginger may also be useful for brain health. Early studies have found the compounds in ginger may protect the brain from Alzheimer's disease and age-related decline. Gotu kola may help boost cognitive function. It should not be used continuously. In Chinese medicine gotu kola is commonly used to treat pathologies associated with heat. Gotu kola is to be used with caution, particularly during pregnancy. Check with your healthcare professional before using.

- 2 gotu kola tea bags
- 1 cup boiling water
- 2 cups vegan milk
- Sweetener to taste
- 2 tablespoons freshly chopped ginger

1. Steep tea bags and ginger in hot water for 10 minutes. Remove tea bags and strain.
2. Place water and milk in a small pot. Heat gently. Add sugar to taste. Enjoy!

LOTUS ROOT FASTING SOUP
Serves 2

To fast is to refrain from eating and/or drinking for a specific period of time. Fasting is normally performed for spiritual purposes or health reasons. There are many ways to fast. Some folks may fast on fruits or liquids. Others may prefer to use only soups, or to eat only one meal daily. Below is a soup made from the lotus root. The lotus is a sacred aquatic flower from the East that grows in muddy swamps, shallow ponds, and flooded fields. Perhaps it is ironic yet fitting that from muddy waters a most beautiful flower blooms.

- 1½ quarts water
- 1 tbsp freshly minced ginger
- ½ medium-size onion, roughly sliced (optional)
- 4 celery stalks, cut into large pieces
- Olive oil and Bragg's liquid aminos to taste
- 2 cups sliced lotus root (sliced to preference—they can be sliced very thinly or into pieces up to ¼ inch wide)
- Freshly ground black pepper to taste (optional)

1. Peel the lotus root. Slice it into ¼ inch slices and quarter.
2. Sauté the onions, ginger, and celery in a small amount of vegetable oil until the herbs are fragrant.
3. Add water, bring the mixture to a simmer, then add the lotus root. Let the mixture simmer for an additional 25 to 40 minutes depending on how soft you prefer your lotus root.
4. Place in two bowls. Strain the soup and use only the liquid if you prefer. Add Bragg's and olive oil to taste.

MUDRAS TO ENHANCE MEDITATIONS

OFFERING GESTURE (VAYAPAK ANJALI MUDRA)

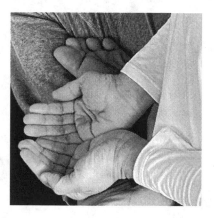

Keeping the shoulders relaxed, let the little finger sides of the palms touch, with the palms cupped and facing forward as though you are offering something to a beloved. Hold for up to 30 minutes as long as the hands are comfortable. This mudra increases one's gratitude, compassion, and generosity.

A HANDFUL OF FLOWERS GESTURE (PUSHPAPUTA MUDRA)

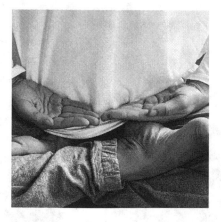

Allow your palms to rest on your lap, palms facing up, thumbs touching the index fingers. This mudra opens us to receiving cosmic consciousness.

MUSIC IDEAS

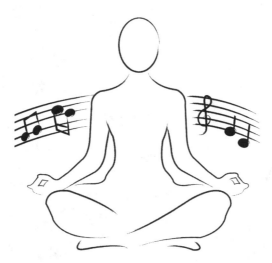

Music that touches the heart and spirit, music of worship, meditative music, music that takes you fully into the present moment.

OTHER BALANCING/STRENGTHENING ACTIVITIES

- Any non-harmful activity that brings you into the present moment
- Prayer
- All forms of meditation
- Practicing acceptance
- Qi gong; tai qi
- Fasting (may be from food or a specific activity)
- Prostrating oneself before one's creator or spiritual deity
- Practicing isvara pranidhana (surrender to a higher power)

Appendix A

Yoga Glossary — Yang Postures

AB-LESS ABDOMINALS WITH A MAT

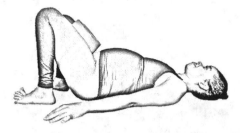

Start lying on the floor with the soles of your feet flat on the floor. Your belly muscles stay relaxed through the entire exercise. Place a rolled-up mat (diameter approximately 8 to 12 inches) between your thighs. Inhale: use your buttock muscles to push your lower back into the floor. Exhale: curl your tailbone up, squeeze your thighs together, and squeeze your sit-bones toward each other (your lower back and buttocks stay on the floor), release. Take a relaxing breath. That is one round. Start with three rounds. As you continue to practice and develop more awareness in this pose, you can do more repetitions.

BAKASANA

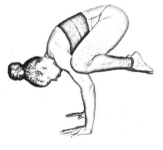

Begin in a squat. Place your hands flat on the floor, slightly closer than shoulders' distance apart. Spread your fingers as much as possible and press your hands firmly down, lift your heels off the floor if they are not off already, and rest your shins on your upper arms. Round your midback toward the ceiling. Pull your belly in. Lift one foot, then the other, off the floor. If you can, lift both feet off the floor. Your neck stays relaxed. Stay in the pose for a few breaths.

BIRTHING SQUAT

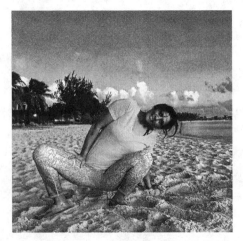

Come into a squat with the feet anywhere from a few inches to just over 1 foot apart. Lean over to your right side; rest your right hand on the floor either in front or behind your hips, or rest your right hand on a block. Place your left hand close to the crease where your left thigh and left hip meet. Press the heel of your left hand down into your left quads and press your quads muscles away from your hips, creating space in your left hip joint. Hold for as long as interests you. Release and repeat on the opposite side. You may choose to spend one breath on each side, alternating between your sides a couple of times. Breathe into your belly, pelvis, groin, and lower back.

BRIDGE

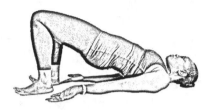

Start on your back, with your legs bent, your feet flat on the floor. Your feet are parallel and slightly wider than your hips' distance apart. Your heels are under your knees. Ease your shoulder blades down your back. Relax your arms by your sides. Inhale: lift your ribcage toward your chin. Exhale: press down through your feet, tuck your tailbone up, and lift your pelvis up. Keep your neck and jaw relaxed. Stay for 5 to 8 breaths in the pose. Focus on first feeling your legs, then your hips, belly, lower back, ribs, and neck. Feel all the chakra territories while in this pose. To release, tuck your tailbone, then slowly lower your upper back, midback, lower back, and then hips onto the mat. If you are practicing Bridge with a Roll, place a roll (approximately 8 inches in diameter) between your thighs close to your pelvis. Lightly squeeze on the roll as you hold the pose. To perform Supported Bridge, place a block at its medium or tall height (if possible) under the sacrum. There should be no pain in your lower back in any of these variations.

CAMEL WITH A ROLL

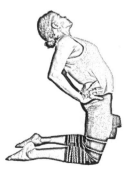

Stand on your knees. Have padding under your shins. Place a roll (approximately 8 inches in diameter) between your thighs, close to your crotch. Squeeze the roll with your inner thighs. Press your shins into the mat and tuck your tailbone down; your sit-bones move toward the roll. Rest your hands on your lower back. Inhale: lift your ribs, arch your chest. Exhale: pull your belly in and keep a strong tuck in the tailbone. Keep your lower back long and pain free. Stay for 3 to 8 breaths in the pose. Focus on making each inhale an exploration into your heart. To release, tuck the tailbone strongly and lift the chest back to a neutral position.

CLASSICAL SPINAL TWIST

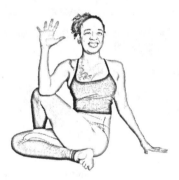

Start in a seated position. Pad your hip or hips if necessary. Bend your right knee and place your right foot by your left hip; your right outer thigh is on the floor. If this is too intense you can practice with your right leg straight. Bring your left foot over your right thigh; your left knee is up. Inhale: lift your chest away from your belly. Exhale: twist to your left, wrap your right arm around your left shin, or place your right elbow to the outside of your knee. Your left arm is on the floor behind your back. Inhale: lengthen your spine upward toward the ceiling. Your hips are firmly grounded. Exhale: keep lifting your spine while relaxing your shoulder blades down away from your ears. Stay for 5 to 8 breaths. Repeat on the opposite side.

COBRA OVER A ROLL

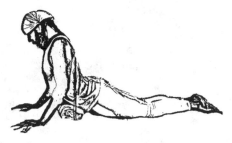

Begin on hands and knees. Rest a roll (approximately 8 inches in diameter) under your navel. You can use a rolled-up mat or blanket for this exercise. Use whatever is most comfortable for your body. Ensure the roll is pressing into your belly, not your ribs. Rest for about 3 breaths over the roll, allowing the roll to come into and massage your belly. Place your hands approximately 1 foot in front of your shoulders. Tuck your tailbone, reach through your legs, and on your inhale lift your chest up and toward your fingertips. On your exhale keep a tuck in your tailbone and lower your ribs down to the floor. Invite the roll into your tummy as you release. This pose is contraindicated in pregnancy or for persons suffering with severe abdominal disorders.

DOLPHIN

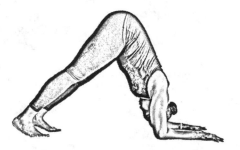

Start on your hands and knees. Bring your elbows down onto the mat and clasp your upper arms. Wrap your fingers around your upper arms. This helps you to find the correct distance for your elbows. On stronger days, work the forearms parallel. On weaker days, work with the hands clasped. Choose your arm position, press your forearms down into the mat, and flex your chest muscles. On your exhale curl your toes under and straighten your legs as much as possible. Press your heels toward the mat. Inhale: spread your ribs. Exhale: lift the shoulders away from the floor, relax your neck and jaw. Stay for 3 to 8 breaths.

DOWNWARD-FACING DOG

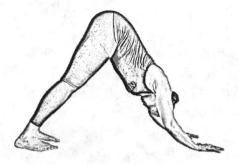

Begin on your hands and knees. Your hands are shoulders' distance apart. Spread your fingers wide apart and press the inner sides of your hands firmly down onto your mat; your wrists are parallel to the front edge of your mat. On an exhale curl your toes under and lift your hips and your knees off the floor. Reach your hips back toward your heels. Your body is in the shape of an inverted 'V.' Completely relax your neck and throat.

EASY TWISTING WARRIOR

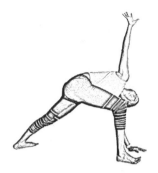

From Downward-Facing Dog step your left leg up between your hands. Turn the right foot down to the left so the right foot is flat on the floor, or stay up on the right toes. With your right hand on the floor or on a block approximately 1 foot away from the inner left ankle, inhale and reach your left hand up to the ceiling. If you are pregnant the right hand should be around 2 feet from the inner left ankle, so that there is no pressure on the baby. Exhale and relax the neck. Inhale: arch the chest toward the inner left thigh. Exhale: reach up and back through your left hand. Stay for a few breaths, opening the chest with your inhales. Repeat on the opposite side.

ELBOW TO KNEE

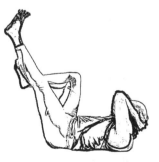

Start with your back flat on the mat (pad the back for comfort). Lift your feet off the floor. Your feet are lower than your knees; your knees are aligned over your pelvis. Inhale: curl your head and shoulders up (elbows reaching toward the ceiling), press your lower back down, curl your tailbone up. Exhale: reach both elbows toward your left knee, straighten your right leg (right heel approximately 3 feet from the floor), pull your belly in. Inhale: come back to center, bend both legs, press your lower back down, curl your tailbone up. Exhale: reach both elbows toward your right knee, straighten your left leg, pull your belly down. That's one round. Do between three and eight rounds. Embrace the sensations in your abdomen.

EXTENDED WARRIOR VARIATION (WITH NECK RELEASE)

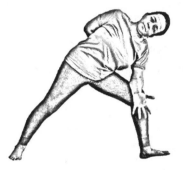

Start in a Warrior 2 position with your left leg forward. Rest your left forearm on your left thigh. Inhale: lift your ribs. Exhale: move your right hand behind your back, grab hold of your left thigh or clothing behind your back. Stay connected to your feet. Inhale: push the left forearm down on the thigh to lift your chest up, away from the thigh. Exhale: relax your neck down toward your left shoulder or (depending on the tightness in your neck) toward the floor. Exhale: draw both shoulder blades down your back, pull belly in, tuck your tailbone. Stay for a few breaths, then repeat on the opposite side.

FORWARD FOLD (WITH NECK TRACTION)

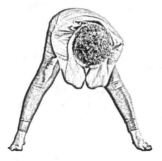

Start in mountain pose. Open your feet at least hips' distance apart. Exhale: pull your belly in and lower your upper body toward the floor. Head relaxed down. Grab hold of two handfuls of hair at the crown of your head and slowly and gently on your exhale pull your head toward the floor. Alternatively, interlock your fingers at the base of the skull and bring your elbows to touch each other; your forearms are under your jawline. Look at the floor. Keep your elbows touching. On your exhale send your elbows slowly down toward the floor beneath your face. Breathe into the sensations in your upper back and neck.

FROG LIFTING THROUGH ABDOMINALS

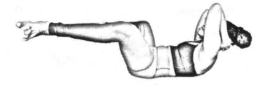

Start with your back flat on the mat (pad the back for comfort). Lift your feet off the floor. Bend your legs to a 90-degree angle and flex your feet. Straddle your legs, open your knees wide apart, knees aligned with your pelvis. Feet turned out. Inhale: curl your head and shoulders up. On your exhale, curl your pubic bone toward your navel, reach out through your thighs, then pull your belly down. Release your pelvis, then inhale into your lower back. Exhale: curl pubic bone toward navel, reach out through thighs, pull belly down. That's two reps. Repeat 1 to 6 times more. Release the head and shoulders to the floor. Place hands on the outer thighs and use your hands to help bring your legs together. Feet down.

HALF MOON

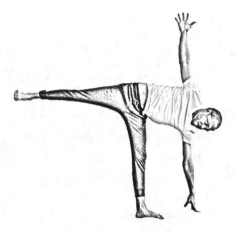

Start in Triangle pose with the left foot turned out 90 degrees, the right foot turning in slightly. Your left hand rests on your left shin. Bend your left leg. Set your left hand down, either on the floor or on a block approximately 5 inches to the outside of the left foot and 12 inches in front of it. Shift the weight into the left hand and pick your right foot off the floor. Reach your right foot back. Reach your right hand up to the ceiling. Imagine a wall behind you—both shoulders, your back, hips, and right heel would be touching that wall. Relax your neck. Stay for 3 to 10 breaths. Repeat on the opposite side.

HEAD TO ANKLE PREPARATION

Start with your feet approximately 4 feet apart, left leg forward in a Warrior 2 stance. On your exhale pull your belly in and rest your hands on the floor under your shoulders or onto a block. Place your left hand on your inner left thigh close to where your thigh and pelvis meet. The right hand is approximately 1 foot to the inside of the right toes. Inhale and arch your chest toward the right. On your exhale push the heel of your left hand into the left thigh; traction the inner thigh muscles away from the pelvis. Breathe into your lower back, hips, and groin. Find sweetness in the pose.

HEADSTAND

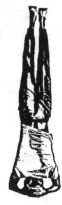

As a safety precaution, practice Headstand first with a qualified teacher. Build sufficient strength through the shoulders to keep the neck long while practicing. Stay focused on each breath.

HORSE STANCE

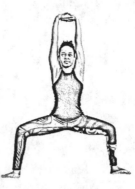

Stand with your feet 3 to 3½ feet apart. Turn your feet out slightly. Bend your knees until your thighs are parallel to the floor and your heels are directly under your knees. Your feet are active; press the balls and heels of your feet strongly into the floor while lifting your toes off the floor. Inhale: lift your ribs. Exhale: lengthen your tailbone down. Horse Stance can be practiced with several different arm variations, for example shoulder shrugs, hand passes, eagle arms, archer arms, birdwing, and unlocking the shoulders.

SEATED SIDE BEND, ONE LEG STRAIGHT WITH CHEST OPENER

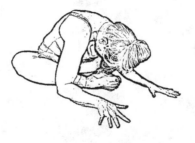

Start seated. Straighten your left leg and bring your right foot in front of your groin. Your thighs are as wide apart as you can comfortably have them. Your chest is in between your thighs. Inhale: reach your left arm straight up to the sky; exhale: place your left hand or left forearm on the floor next to the inner left thigh. Inhale: reach your right arm straight up to the sky; exhale: move the right hand 2 to 3 inches toward your right hip, then reach your right arm back to open across the front of your chest. Inhale: arch your chest. Exhale: relax the neck; your right shoulder blade moves down the back. Inhale into the opening in the chest. Stay for 5 to 10 breaths, then repeat on the opposite side.

SEATED SIDE BEND, ONE LEG STRAIGHT WITH NECK RELEASE

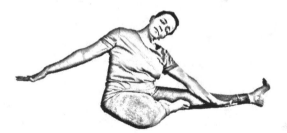

Start seated. Straighten your left leg and bring your right foot in front of your groin. The thighs are as wide apart as you can comfortably have them. Your chest is in between your thighs. Inhale: reach your left arm up; exhale: place your left hand or left forearm on the floor next to the inner left thigh. Reach your right hand back, so your right hand is a few inches away from the floor. Reach through your right arm to help lengthen your neck. Release your neck down over your left shoulder as you reach your right hand away from your shoulder. Inhale: arch your chest. Exhale: relax your neck; your mouth can open slightly. Stay for 5 to 10 breaths, then repeat on the opposite side.

SHOULDERSTAND

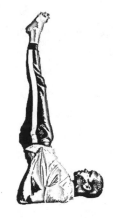

As a safety precaution, practice Shoulderstand first with a qualified teacher. Many students need to support the neck and shoulders with padding when practicing Shoulderstand. You may want to try Bridge at the Wall which involves coming into Bridge pose close to the wall (pad the shoulders and the lower half of the neck with padding). Step one foot up the wall and then the other. This is a modified Shoulderstand position from which students can experiment with taking one foot, then both feet, off the wall. The neck and jaw should be relaxed in Shoulderstand. Focus on your breathing in the pose.

SUN SALUTATIONS

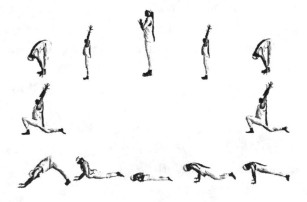

Start standing in mountain pose. Exhale: place your hands into namaste. Inhale: reach your hands to the sky, your fingers spread wide apart; lift your ribs. Exhale: pull your belly in and fold forward; your hands rest on the floor on either side of your feet or onto blocks. Relax your head down to the floor. Inhale: step your left leg back into a lunge position, back knee down on the floor; reach your hands up to the ceiling. Exhale: place both hands on the floor. Inhale: move into plank pose / upper pushup position. Exhale: lower your torso to the floor. Draw your shoulders down away from your ears as you lower to the floor. Tuck your tailbone, reach back through your legs, press hands into the floor. Inhale: lift your chest into Cobra. Exhale: move into Downward-Facing Dog. Inhale: step your left foot in between your hands into lunge. Exhale: step your right foot forward into a standing forward bend. Inhale: reach up into mountain pose. Exhale: place your hands into namaste. With a focus on the third chakra, you can move quickly (while keeping good form in the pose). You can also embrace and be enlivened by the heat the Sun Salutations create in the body. With a focus on the seventh chakra, savor being present in each aspect of the flow. Tune in to as much sensation as you can while moving with grace.

TREE

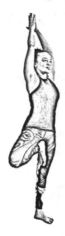

Start standing. Shift your weight onto your left hip and foot. The right leg feels light. Plant the ball and heel of your left foot into the floor. Feel the inner and outer edges of your left foot pressing into the floor. Place your right foot along your inner leg, below or above your knee. On your inhale reach your hands to the ceiling. As you exhale continue to focus on grounding your left foot into the floor.

TRIANGLE

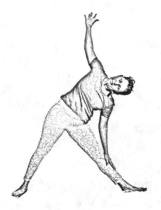

From mountain pose, open your feet approximately 3 feet apart; the feet are parallel to each other. Turn your left foot out 90 degrees and turn your right foot in slightly. The left heel is aligned to the arch of your right foot. Inhale: lift your chest. Inhale: lift your arms out to shoulder height. Exhale: reach your left arm out over your left leg; let your left hand rest on the left leg. The right hand reaches up to the sky. Relax your neck. Imagine a wall behind you—both shoulders, your back, and your hips would be touching that wall. Hold for 3 to 8 breaths. Repeat on the opposite side.

TWISTING HORSE STANCE

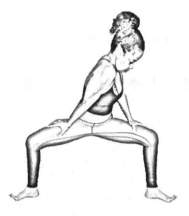

Stand with your feet 3 to 3½ feet apart. Turn your feet out slightly. Bend your legs until your knees are directly over your heels. Place your hands on top of your thighs a few inches away from your knees. On your exhale, bend and twist toward your left knee. Your right arm is straight. Your right hand is pushing against your right thigh. Inhale: expand your ribs and lengthen your torso away from your hips. On your exhale, relax your neck. Stay grounded through the feet as you breathe in a way that feels pleasurable in the pose.

WARRIOR 1

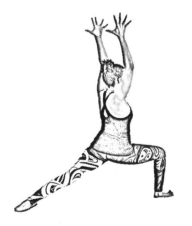

Start standing, with your feet approximately 3 to 4 feet apart. Turn your left foot out 90 degrees. Turn your right foot in approximately 60 degrees. Your left heel is aligned with your right heel. Move the left foot more to the left if you feel unstable in the pose. Your hips are parallel to the front edge of your mat. Plant both feet firmly into the mat. On your exhale, bend your left knee. Inhale: reach your arms up to the sky. Inhale: lift your ribs. Exhale and feel your feet like roots connecting down into the earth.

Yoga Glossary—Yin Postures

Please note that the instructions given in this section are meant to be guidelines for the execution of the postures. Our bodies are all different and as such your poses will be unique to you.

BABY DRAGON

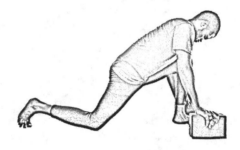

From either hands and knees or Downward-Facing Dog, step one foot between your hands. Ease the front foot forward until the knee is directly above your ankle. Keep your hands on either side of the front foot. You can rest your hands either on blocks or on the floor, depending on the sensations in your body.

BANANASANA

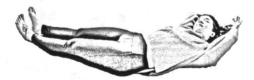

Start on your back, on the floor with your legs together. Move your legs over to the right (while keeping your left buttock grounded) and move your head and chest over to the right, creating a banana shape with your body. If you like, you can cross the ankles to intensify the posture. Find a comfortable position for your arms. The arms may be overhead as pictured, or reach the left arm down away from the shoulder to create a stretch in the neck.

CATERPILLAR

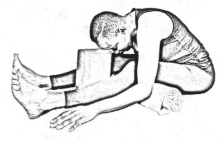

Start sitting in staff pose, with your legs straight. Open the legs anywhere from a few inches to hips' width apart. Lean forward. Allow the weight of your head and upper body to relax toward the floor. This pose can be practiced with props under the knees if the sensations in the back and hamstrings are too intense, and with a block or cushions under the forehead to draw awareness to the third eye.

CHILD'S POSE

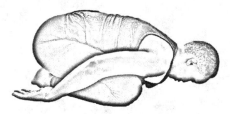

Start on your hands and shins. Move your hips back and allow your ribs to rest on top of or toward your thighs. Your hands can be stretched forward or by your sides. There should be only mild to moderate sensations in the pose. No pain in the joints. If there is pain in the knees try placing a blanket behind the knees, between your thighs and knees. Have the ankles on padding if necessary. Allow the weight of the head to settle into or toward the floor. If the sensations are still too intense, avoid the pose or practice knee-to-chest pose with your back on the floor, drawing your knees in toward your chest.

DANGLING

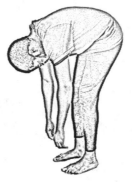

Start standing. Softly bend your knees. Inhale, and on your exhale release your upper body down into a forward fold. Let your neck, jaw, and throat relax. Clasp your elbows and allow the weight of your arms to relax toward the floor. Depending on the sensations in your body, you may want to rest your elbows on your thighs or let your arms dangle toward the floor. Stay connected to the sensations in your legs, lower back, pelvis, and feet. Stay grounded through the inner and outer edges of your feet.

DRAGON FLYING HIGH

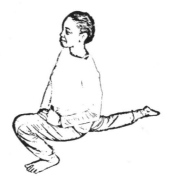

From either hands and knees or Downward-Facing Dog, step your left foot between your hands. Ease the left foot forward until the left knee is directly above your left heel. Lift your chest and rest your hands on your left thigh. Press both feet gently down into the floor. Sometimes you may want to focus on lifting the weight of the chest up on your inhales. Depending on your flexibility, the front knee may extend over your left foot. Stay for a few breaths, then change sides.

FIRE-BREATHING DRAGON (DRAGON FLYING LOW)

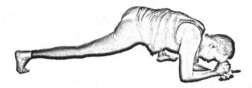

From either hands and knees or Downward-Facing Dog, step your left foot between your hands. Ease the left foot forward until the left knee is directly above your left heel. Place both hands on the inside of your left foot. More flexible students can bring their forearms onto the floor and their hips closer to the floor. Working with the back knee up is known as Fire-Breathing Dragon. With the back knee down, the pose is known as Dragon Flying Low. Keep relaxing your head down throughout your stay in the pose. There is little to no tension in your shoulders. Repeat on the opposite leg.

HALF HAPPY BABY

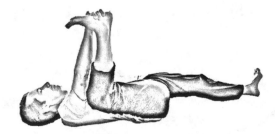

Start lying on your back with both legs bent, your feet flat on the floor. Hug your left foot into your chest, then grab the sole of the left foot, left ankle, or back of the left leg with your left hand. You may also use a strap if that makes the pose more accessible to you. Have your left ankle, if possible, above the left knee. If sensations will permit, straighten your right leg. Breathe into the belly, lower back, and hips.

HEART-MELTING POSE

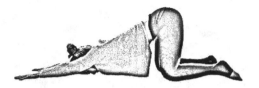

Begin on your hands and knees. Spread your fingers wide; have your hands parallel to the front edge of your mat. Move your knees back approximately 1 foot and allow your chest to melt toward the floor. Rest your knees on extra padding if you like. Your hips are directly over your knees. Breathe in a way that opens your chest and heart.

RECLINING DEER

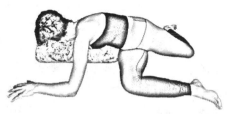

Start in a seated position. Take your right leg behind your hips and move your left leg, if possible, into a 90-degree angle or as close to a 90-degree angle as you comfortably can. Have a bolster or cushions next to your left hip. Slowly lower your upper body to rest on your cushions or bolsters. Your hands are on either side of your props. Your head is turned either toward your right or your left. There is no pain in the knees; the sensations in your body are mild to moderate. If the sensations in Deer pose are too intense or if the pose is not accessible to you, omit it.

RECLINING SUPPORTED BUTTERFLY

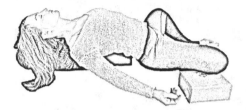

In a seated position, bring the soles of your feet to touch; your legs form a diamond shape. Support your outer thighs with blocks if you prefer. Lie down, resting your back on support; use either pillows, bolsters, or blocks. Breathe in a way that gently lifts your sternum and front ribs. More advanced students: breathe into your heart.

RECLINING TWIST

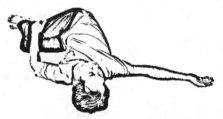

Start lying on your back with your knees drawn in toward your chest; your feet are off the floor. Move your arms straight out from the shoulders, palms down. If there is tingling in the arms or hands or extreme discomfort in the shoulders (listen to your body), lower the arms from parallel to the shoulders or rest them on your ribs. The symptoms should abate. Drop your knees to one side of your body. Play with the knee position; having your knees closer or further away from your shoulders changes the effect of the pose on your spine. Breathe into the bottom-most area of your ribcage.

SADDLE

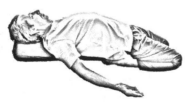

Start on hands and knees. You can either sit on or in between your heels. You may need to sit on props (such as blocks) that are placed between your feet. If there is pain in your knees, omit this posture. Instead lie on your belly, head resting on a forearm, and using your hand or a strap, draw one foot in toward the buttocks. For those who can sit comfortably, lean back onto your hands. Perhaps you can rest on your forearms or a bolster (or pillows), perhaps you cannot lean back which is OK. Remember you are aiming for mild to moderate sensations in your back and a mild to moderate stretch in your quadricep muscles. Breathe into the bottom-most area of your ribcage or where in your core you are feeling a compression or a stretch.

SAVASANA

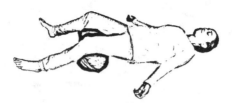

Lie on the floor. You may be able to relax the body more by resting with a bolster or cushions under your knees. Use each inhale to draw your attention to a specific part of your body, for example your feet. Use each exhale to release the weight of that part of your body into the floor beneath you. Sometimes it may take more than one breath to relax an area. Do what helps you to relax the most. Once you have relaxed your body, notice the stillness and heaviness in your body. Stay present to that sensation. Stay connected to the flow of your breath. This is but one way to practice savasana.

SEATED BUTTERFLY

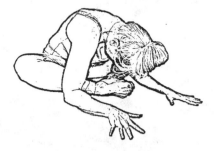

Sit on a cushion or the floor, depending on your flexibility. Bring the soles of your feet to touch each other. Depending on how much sensation you want in the pose, move your heels either away or toward your groin. Remember the intensity in yin yoga postures should be no more than mild to moderate. Inhale, and on your exhale fold forward, easing your chest and head toward the floor. Allow your shoulders and arms to relax. Work with blocks under your outer knees if you feel you need the extra support. You can also rest the head on a block or cushions.

SEATED NECK RELEASE

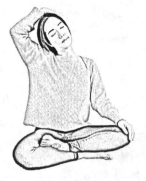

From a seated position, release your head to your left side. You can open your jaw slightly and rest your tongue on the roof of your mouth. You may also want to rest your left hand on top of your right ear to deepen the stretch in the neck. You are not pulling on the neck, only allowing the weight of the left hand to deepen the stretch. Repeat on the opposite side.

SEATED SPINAL TWIST

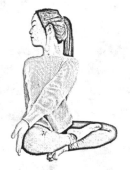

Start in a comfortable seated position. Inhale: lift your ribs away from your diaphragm and sit tall. Exhale: twist to your left; your right hand rests on your left knee; left hand rests on the floor behind you. Inhale: continue to gently lift your ribs. Exhale: relax your shoulder blades down your back. There is very little to no tension in the arms or hands. Either stay with your head in a neutral position or slowly look toward your left or right shoulder. Allow the tongue to rest on the roof of the mouth; you can also open the mouth slightly to help relax the jaw.

SPHINX (AND WIDE-LEG SPHINX)

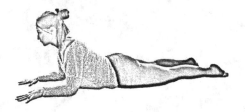

Begin lying on your belly. Lift up onto your elbows. Your forearms are parallel to each other; your elbows are under your shoulders. If the sensations in your back are too intense you may want to ease the elbows forward. You can intensify the pose by resting your forearms on a bolster or blocks. Breathe into your chest. In Wide-Leg Sphinx the legs are open at least hip distance apart or wider. Opening the legs into Wide-Leg Sphinx is sometimes more comfortable.

STRADDLE (SIDE BEND VARIATION)

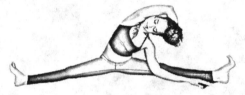

Start in a seated position on the floor. Open your legs as wide apart as you comfortably can. Lean over to your right. Your right hand or right forearm is resting on the floor to the inside of the right thigh. Inhale and reach your left hand over your ears. For a more dynamic stretch in the arm, reach your left finger toward your right toe; otherwise allow the left arm to rest lightly against the head. Stay for at least 90 seconds, then switch sides.

SWAN

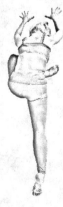

From Downward-Facing Dog or hands and knees, step your left foot forward and ease your left foot toward your right hand. Rest on your outer left thigh. Your left foot may be close to the pelvis or your left leg may be bent at a 90-degree angle. Choose a leg position that allows you to center your weight if possible. Notice the amount of sensation in your hips and knees; remember the sensations should be mild to moderate. Stay in the pose with the chest lifted for more of a backbend, or release the chest and head down toward the floor for Sleeping Swan. If the sensations in the knees are too intense, practice instead a Reclining Figure Four pose. In Reclining Figure Four pose, your back is on the floor. Start with both feet flat on the floor. Cross the left foot over the right thigh and then draw the right thigh in toward your chest.

TOE SQUAT

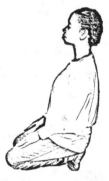

Begin standing on your shins. Curl your toes under. Sit back onto your heels. Focus on the feelings of your body in the pose. Allow those sensations to keep you fully in the present. Stay only for a few breaths or for as long as the sensations remain mild to moderate. Don't stay in the pose if it is painful or the sensations are too intense. Some yogis take mini breaks in the Toe Squat when it becomes too challenging by standing on the shins (the starting position).

TWISTING HALF BUTTERFLY

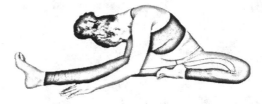

Start seated, either on a cushion or on the floor. Draw one foot in toward your groin and stretch the other leg straight out to the side. Twist your torso toward either the bent or straight leg. Inhale, and on your exhale ease into a forward fold over either the bent or straight leg. Allow your shoulders and arms to relax. Allow your head to relax down toward the floor. Work with a block under the knee of the bent leg if you feel you need the extra support. You can rest your head on a block or cushions.

WALL CATERPILLAR (MODIFIED)

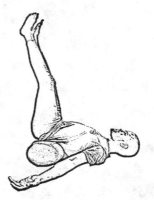

Lie on your back with your legs up the wall. Have your pelvis higher than your shoulders by supporting your pelvis with bolsters or cushions. Ease your shoulders away from your ears. Allow the weight of your legs to rest on the wall. There should be no discomfort in your lower back. Aim for a mild to moderate stretch through the back of the legs. Focus on the sensations in your legs. If the sensations are too intense, try moving the hips a few inches away from the wall. If possible, stay for at least 5 minutes or more.

WALL STRADDLE

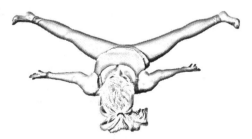

Start lying on your back with your legs up the wall (Wall Caterpillar). Straddle your legs. As you stay in the pose, gravity will draw the legs apart. You may want to rest the outer thighs on blocks to allow for more leg and hip support.

Appendix C

Yoga Glossary — Terms

ACUPOINTS

Acupoints, short for "acupuncture points," are points on the surface of the body which when stimulated can affect our physical, emotional, and mental well-being. Most acupoints belong to the 14 main meridians of the body. The effectiveness of an acupoint for treating poor health depends on several different factors. Though some acupoints are powerful enough on their own to elicit a change in the well-being of a person, acupuncturists will normally needle a group of acupoints to create well-being.

AFFIRMATIONS

Affirmations are positive statements repeated often, either aloud or in our heads. Affirmations can help us challenge and overcome negative thoughts. Affirmations are believed to be more powerful when they are tailored specifically to our life situations and are truly believable to us.

AGNI SARA

The Sanskrit phrase *agni sara* translates to mean 'fire essence.' Agni sara is an advanced yogic practice that involves contracting and releasing the abdomen after an exhalation. It is used by yogis to improve digestive health and enhance overall health. Agni sara should be learned from a qualified yoga practitioner.

AHIMSA

A Sanskrit word that means nonviolence: nonviolence toward all life as well as oneself.

AJNA

Ajna is the Sanskrit word for the brow or third eye chakra. It is located along the central energy channel, level with the top of the spinal column. In twentieth-century yoga, ajna is associated with the color indigo, the pituitary gland (or sometimes the pineal gland), the musical note A, and the planet Neptune. Key words associated with this chakra include vision, perception, and wisdom. It is commonly depicted as a two-petaled lotus. It is also associated with the intuitive and intellectual archetypes.

ANAHATA

Anahata is the Sanskrit word for the heart chakra. The heart chakra is located in the center of the central energy line of our body, approximately level with the xiphoid process of the sternum. In twentieth-century yoga, anahata is associated with the colors green (its primary color) and pink, the heart muscle, the musical note F, and the planet Venus. Key words associated with this chakra are love, kindness, and compassion. It is commonly depicted as a twelve- or ten-petaled lotus. It is also associated with the lover and actor archetypes.

APARIGRAHA

A Sanskrit word that means freedom from hoarding or collecting. It can be translated to mean 'non-possessiveness' or 'non-grasping.'

ASTRAGALUS ROOT

Astragalus root (*Astragali radix / Astragalus membranaceus*) is an adaptogenic herb that has been used for centuries in Traditional Chinese Medicine to boost immunity, reduce edema, relieve numbness and pain, and so on. It can be bought in tea or herb form in most Asian supermarkets, some healthfood stores, and at large online retailers.

CHAKRA

In traditional tantric yoga, chakras are focal points for meditation in the body. These focal points are located over areas of the body where energy can be strongly felt. In traditional tantric yoga there are several different chakra systems, each system containing its own specific number of chakras. In twentieth-century Western yoga, chakras are defined as spinning disks of light, vortexes of energy or energy centers that sit on a central energy channel located along the vertical axis of the body. The chakras of twentieth-century Western yoga are associated with specific psychological states.

CONGENITAL ENERGY

Congenital energy is the energy we are born with. We receive our congenital energy from our parents. Congenital energy determines to some extent our physical and mental health and our ability to reproduce.

DANTIAN

Dantian is a Chinese word that translates to mean 'elixir field.' An elixir field is an energy center that holds something precious. Dantians are important focal points for meditation in Taoism. In Traditional Chinese Medicine the dantians are considered energy centers (or reservoirs) that store the vital substances necessary for life. There are three dantians within the human body. Each dantian is associated with a specific vital substance. The lower dantian stores essence, the middle dantian stores qi, and the upper dantian houses the mind or spirit.

DUALITY OF LIFE

This term is used to describe our present earthly existence in which yin and yang, and good and evil, exist together to create a complete whole. Every aspect of life is created from a balanced interaction of opposite, competing, yet complementary forces.

EARTHING

Earthing (also known as grounding) is the practice of making a physical connection between the body and the earth's surface. Earthing is performed by walking barefoot, sitting, or lying on the earth's surface while wearing organic clothing, or by using conductive mats and blankets, that transfer the energy of the earth to the human body. Research is finding that earthing has several benefits. It is purportedly useful for chronic stress, inflammation, insomnia, pain, and other conditions. It has been suggested that sleeping while earthing will give the best results. However, 30 minutes of earthing daily is also believed to be beneficial for health.

EMBODYING SPIRIT

Embodying spirit is a practice found in Forrest yoga that involves enlivening the entire body using the breath and intent. The objective of this practice is to make the physical body a safe and welcoming residence for our spirit.

ENERGETIC BODY

The aspect of our being that is considered more subtle than the physical body. In Chinese medicine it includes the meridians, the five spirits (each one associated with a specific organ), and the dantian. In some yoga traditions it includes the chakras and nadis (channels through which subtle energies and blood flow).

ESSENCE

The fundamental building block of our physical body. Essence is given to us by our parents and to some extent from our foods. Essence determines our overall health, vitality, stamina, life span, and our ability to reproduce. It is considered the most concentrated yin qi of our body.

GINSENG

The name 'ginseng' is used today to refer to several different herbs. The recipe in this book uses American or Canadian ginseng (*Panax quinquefolium*). Be certain to check the pharmaceutical and/or botanical name before purchasing. American ginseng can be found in most Chinese supermarkets and at online retailers such as Amazon. Asian (Chinese/Korean) ginseng is another form of ginseng commonly used today for medicinal purposes. Asian ginseng (*Panax ginseng* or *Radix ginseng*) is stronger than American ginseng and is used to warm the body and boost energy. Asian ginseng, however, is not suitable for certain persons or for long-term use. Both types of ginseng are known as adaptogens in Western medicine. Please check with your healthcare practitioner before supplementing with any form of ginseng.

GOJI BERRIES

Goji berries (*Lycii fructus*), also known as Chinese wolfberries or lycium fruit, are small red fruits native to Asia. They are commonly sold dried and can be found in most Western healthfood stores and at large online retailers. In their dried form, goji berries are similar to raisins in shape. Look for bright red fruit when purchasing. Check with your healthcare provider before using; goji berries may trigger allergic reactions in some persons and may also interact with certain drugs.

GOTU KOLA

Gotu kola (*Centella asiatica*) is an herb in the parsley family. It is also known as Indian or Asiatic pennywort. Gotu kola is sold in loose form or as tea bags in healthfood stores or at large online retailers. Please check with your healthcare provider before supplementing with this herb.

INTERMITTENT FASTING

Intermittent fasting is an eating pattern that cycles between periods of fasting and eating. Intermittent fasting includes several different eating patterns. Three popular forms of intermittent fasting are: Time Restricted Eating which includes the 16/8 method (fasting for 16 hours daily and eating and/or drinking for only 8 hours daily); the Eat Stop Eat method (fasting for 24 hours once or more weekly); and the 5:2 diet (eating normally for 5 days weekly, then restricting calories to 500 or 600 calories on the remaining 2 days of the week). Health benefits associated with intermittent fasting include weight loss, improved brain and heart health, reduced inflammation, cancer prevention, and reduced insulin resistance. Always check with your healthcare provider before starting any new healthcare programs.

INTUITIVE ABILITY

The ability to know things without having to use conscious reasoning.

ISVARA PRANIDHANA

Isvara is a Sanskrit word that translates to mean 'supreme being,' 'god,' or 'true self.' *Pranidhana* translates to mean 'fixing.' *Isvara pranidhana* can be translated to mean 'fixing oneself or the true self,' or 'dedicating oneself to a supreme being.'

LOTUS ROOT

Lotus root is the underwater rhizome of the aquatic plant *Nelumbo nucifera*. It is the edible root of the lotus flower. It is eaten raw or cooked, and it can be purchased in most Asian groceries. Look for fresh roots that are firm, light brown, and free of cracks, soft spots, or blemishes.

MANIPURA

Manipura is the Sanskrit word for the solar plexus chakra in Western yoga. The solar plexus chakra is located on the central energy channel below the heart chakra at the level of the navel. In twentieth-century yoga, manipura is associated with the color yellow, the pancreas, the musical note E, and the sun. Key words associated with this chakra include expansion, energy, and will. Manipura is commonly depicted as a 10- or 12-petaled lotus. It is also associated with the warrior and servant archetypes.

MASA

Masa is a nixtamalized corn flour. Nixtamalization is a traditional preparation, believed to have been created by the Aztecs, where grain is cooked and soaked in an alkaline solution. Look for masa in Latin/Mexican supermarkets and at large online retailers.

MERIDIAN

A meridian is an energetic pathway or channel within the body through which qi and blood moves. Meridians are located deep within the body as well as superficially. Meridians connect the entire body, as well as protect the body. Meridians connect our organs to our skin, other organs, and our primary sources of vitality. Meridians can be compared to rivers; rivers within the body that circulate the vital substances necessary for life.

MOTHER POINT

Mother points are also known as tonification or reinforcing acupoints. Mother points in general are used to nurture and nourish their associated organ and meridian. Each of the 12 major meridians has a mother point. In the Five Element Theory, each organ of the body is associated with a specific element and each element has a mother element and a son element. Mother points can also be used to nourish their son meridian and/or organ as well.

MUDRA

A mudra is a seal or sealing posture. Yogis believe that mudras influence the qi or prana (life force energy) that flows through the body. There are body mudras and hand mudras.

MULADHARA

Muladhara is the Sanskrit word for the root chakra. The root chakra in Western yoga sits at the bottom of the central energy channel in our body. The central energy channel runs from the top of our head to our pelvic floor. Muladhara is located in the pelvic region above the anus, close to the coccyx. In twentieth-century yoga, muladhara is associated with the colors red (its primary color) and black, the adrenals, the musical note C, and the planet Saturn. Key words associated with this chakra in Western yoga include awakening, matter, survival, and self-preservation. It is commonly depicted as a four-petaled lotus. Muladhara is also associated with the mother and victim archetypes.

NAULI

Nauli is a kriya or cleansing process that involves moving the abdominal muscles in a surging motion. Nauli massages the abdomen. It is used by some yoga practitioners for its health benefits. It is considered particularly useful to improve digestive health. Nauli is an advanced yogic exercise. It should be learned from a qualified yoga practitioner.

NONDUALITY

Nonduality refers to a state of pure awareness considered in many religions to be the fundamental principle of God.

Recognition of this nondual state involves understanding that underlying all existence is a single, infinite awareness from which all things (such as thoughts, emotions and molecules) are derived.

PHYSICAL BODY

The physical body is the densest and most material aspect of our existence. It consists of atoms, molecules, and cells that join together to create for example organs, connective tissue, and blood. Our physical body is enlivened by our energetic bodies.

PROPRIOCEPTION

Proprioception is our body's ability to sense its location, movement, and actions. Proprioception disorders include issues with balance, uncoordinated movements, poor posture, and difficulties recognizing your own strength.

QI

Qi is a term that is frequently used to describe energy or the 'ability to function' in Traditional Chinese Medicine. A wider understanding of qi considers it the basis of everything in the universe—immaterial and material. Shen or spirit is a form of qi, and essence is also a form of qi. Every organ of the body has its own qi; everything in the universe has its own qi. Having good overall qi and organ qi is vital for good health in Traditional Chinese Medicine.

QI GONG

Qi gong is a Chinese phrase that can be translated to mean 'energy cultivation.' Qi gong, like tai chi, consists of gentle movements designed to improve mental, emotional, and physical health. Tai chi, when practiced for health cultivation, is a form of qi gong.

SAHASRARA

Sahasrara is the Sanskrit word for the crown chakra. In some ancient traditions the crown chakra is not considered a chakra. The crown chakra is located at the top of our central energetic channel, at the top of our head or slightly above it. In twentieth-century yoga it is associated with the colors white, violet, or gold, the pineal gland (sometimes the pituitary gland), the musical note B, and the planet Uranus. Key words associated with this chakra include grace, divinity, true and pure awareness. It is commonly depicted as a thousand-petaled lotus. It is also associated with the guru and egotist archetypes.

SANJIAO

Sanjiao is a concept in Traditional Chinese Medicine that divides the chest and abdomen into three regions. *Sanjiao* translates to mean 'three burners' or 'triple burner.' It is considered an organ in Traditional Chinese Medicine. The sanjiao is made up of three jiaos (burners). The upper jiao is located in the chest region, the middle jiao is located in the abdomen above the navel, and the lower jiao is located in the adomen below the navel.

SANTOSHA

Santosha or *santosa* is a Sanskrit term that can be translated to mean 'completely satisfied,' 'entirely comfortable,' or 'contentment.' Practicing santosha involves a shift from focusing on our desires to accepting and appreciating who we are and what we already have.

SHEN

Shen is a purified form of qi that is often translated to mean spirit, mind, or state of consciousness. The quality of our shen determines our ability to think and reason.

SVADHISTHANA

Svadhisthana is the Sanskrit word for the sacral chakra in Western yoga. The sacral chakra is located directly above muladhara on the central energy channel approximately 2 inches below the navel. In twentieth-century yoga it is associated with the color orange, the gonads, the musical note D, and the planet Pluto. Key words associated with this chakra in Western yoga include self-expression, creativity, sensuality, and rising consciousness. It is commonly depicted as a six-petaled lotus. It is also associated with the emperor/empress and the martyr archetypes.

SVADHYANA

Svadhyana can be defined as the study of self or self-reflection. In many teachings it involves studying sacred texts in order to attain wisdom of the self.

TAI CHI

Tai chi, short for *tai chi chuan*, is a Chinese phrase that means 'supreme ultimate fist.' Tai chi is a soft form of martial arts, a moving meditation that is practiced for defense training and health benefits. Tai chi consists of a series of slow-motion exercises designed to create harmony between the body and mind. Health benefits associated with tai chi include improved strength, flexibility, balance, and coordination.

TAOISM

Taoism or Daoism is a religion and philosophy from ancient China that emphasizes that humans should live in harmony with the Tao, or the universe.

TRADITIONAL CHINESE MEDICINE

Traditional Chinese Medicine is a life science that has been used for thousands of years in China and Asia to create good health. Traditional Chinese Medicine includes the practice of acupuncture, Chinese massage, Chinese herbal medicine, and qi gong. One of the fundamental ideas of Traditional Chinese Medicine is that good health can be achieved and maintained once the energy of our body flows freely and is balanced.

TRATAKA

Trataka is a form of meditation where practitioners gaze steadily at a small object such as a candle flame. This practice should only be attempted under the guidance of an experienced teacher as it is not recommended for all persons.

UDDIYANA

Uddiyana is an advanced breathing exercise in yoga that involves pulling the abdominal muscles in toward the spine and up after an exhalation. Uddiyana is a bandha. A bandha is considered a lock or form of bondage, in which certain parts of the body are contracted. Uddiyana is believed to improve digestive and overall health. Practices such as uddiyana when not learned correctly can damage health. Please seek out the guidance of a qualified practitioner to learn this exercise.

VISHUDDHA

Vishuddha is the Sanskrit word for the throat chakra. The throat chakra is located along the central energetic channel in the throat. In twentieth-century yoga it is associated with the color blue, the thyroid and parathyroid glands, the musical note G, and the planet Mercury. Key words associated with the throat chakra include purification, communication, caution, and expression. It is commonly depicted as a 16-petaled lotus. It is also associated with the communicator and the silent child archetypes.

YANG

A concept in Chinese philosophy used to describe the world in which we live. Everything can be described as either yin or yang. Yang qualities are described as being more active, fast, light, warm, expanding, moving, growing, and masculine. In the body, yang is used to describe the upper, posterior, and exterior parts of the body. Physiologically it represents organ function. Yang is never used without its complement and opposite yin.

YIN

A concept in Chinese philosophy used to describe the world in which we live. Everything can be described as either yin or yang. Yin qualities are described as being more restful, slow, dark, cold, closing, nourishing, contracting, and feminine. In the body, yin is used to describe the lower, anterior, and interior parts of the body. Physiologically it represents the substances of the body, such as blood, saliva, and other body fluids. Yin is never used without its complement and opposite yang.

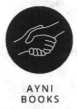

AYNI
BOOKS

ALTERNATIVE HEALTH & HEALING

"Ayni" is a Quechua word meaning "reciprocity" - sharing, giving and receiving - whatever you give out comes back to you. To be in Ayni is to be in balance, harmony and right relationship with oneself and nature, of which we are all an intrinsic part. Complementary and Alternative approaches to health and wellbeing essentially follow a holistic model, within which one is given support and encouragement to move towards a state of balance, true health and wholeness, ultimately leading to the awareness of one's unique place in the Universal jigsaw of life - Ayni, in fact. If you have enjoyed this book, why not tell other readers by posting a review on your preferred book site.

Recent bestsellers from AYNI Books are:

Reclaiming Yourself from Binge Eating
A Step-By-Step Guide to Healing
Leora Fulvio, MFT
Win the war against binge eating, wake up each morning at peace with your body, unafraid of food and overeating.
Paperback: 978-1-78099-680-6 ebook: 978-1-78099-681-3

The Reiki Sourcebook (revised ed.)
Frans Stiene, Bronwen Stiene
A popular, comprehensive and updated manual for the Reiki
novice, teacher and general reader.
Paperback: 978-1-84694-181-8 ebook: 978-1-84694-648-6

The Chakras Made Easy
Hilary H. Carter
From the successful Made Easy series, Chakras Made Easy is a
practical guide to healing the seven chakras.
Paperback: 978-1-78099-515-1 ebook: 978-1-78099-516-8

The Inner Heart of Reiki
Rediscovering Your True Self
Frans Stiene
A unique journey into the inner heart of the system of Reiki,
to help practitioners and teachers rediscover their True Selves.
Paperback: 978-1-78535-055-9 ebook: 978-1-78535-056-6

Middle Age Beauty
Soulful Secrets from a Former Face Model Living Botox Free in
Her Forties
Machel Shull
Find out how to look fabulous during middle age without
plastic surgery by learning inside secrets from a former model.
Paperback: 978-1-78099-574-8 ebook: 978-1-78099-575-5

The Optimized Woman
Using Your Menstrual Cycle to Achieve Success and
Fulfillment
Miranda Gray
If you want to get ahead, get a cycle! For women who want to
create life-success in a female way.
Paperback: 978-1-84694-198-6

The Patient in Room Nine Says He's God
Louis Profeta
A roller coaster ride of joy, controversy, triumph and tragedy;
often all on the same page.
Paperback: 978-1-84694-354-6 ebook: 978-1-78099-736-0

Re-humanizing Medicine
A Holistic Framework for Transforming Your Self, Your
Practice, and the Culture of Medicine
David Raymond Kopacz
Re-humanizing medical practice for doctors, clinicians,
clients, and systems.
Paperback: 978-1-78279-075-4 ebook: 978-1-78279-074-7

**You Can Beat Lung Cancer Using Alternative/Integrative
Interventions**
Carl O. Helvie R.N., Dr.P.H.
Significantly increase your chances of long-term lung
cancer survival by using holistic alternative and integrative
interventions by physicians or health practitioners.
Paperback: 978-1-78099-283-9 ebook: 978-1-78099-284-6

Readers of ebooks can buy or view any of these bestsellers by
clicking on the live link in the title. Most titles are published
in paperback and as an ebook. Paperbacks are available in
traditional bookshops. Both print and ebook formats are
available online.

Find more titles and sign up to our readers' newsletter at
http:// www.johnhuntpublishing.com/mind-body-spirit
Follow us on Facebook at https://www.facebook.com/OBooks
and Twitter at https://twitter.com/obooks